ALLERGY AND ASTHMA
MADE EASY

For my parents, Dr Abdul Sami
and Amtul Rehman Sami

ALLERGY AND ASTHMA
MADE EASY

AMTUL SALAM SAMI

MBBS, BSc, ODTC, MCPS, MA, MSc
Specialist in E.N.T. and Allergy
Lewisham and Greenwich NHS Trust, London

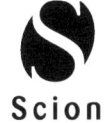

Scion

© **Scion Publishing Ltd, 2020**

ISBN 9781911510352

First published 2020

A CIP catalogue record for this book is available from the British Library.

Scion Publishing Limited

The Old Hayloft, Vantage Business Park, Bloxham Road, Banbury OX16 9UX, UK

www.scionpublishing.com

Important Note from the Publisher

The information contained within this book was obtained by Scion Publishing Ltd from sources believed by us to be reliable. However, while every effort has been made to ensure its accuracy, no responsibility for loss or injury whatsoever occasioned to any person acting or refraining from action as a result of information contained herein can be accepted by the authors or publishers.

Readers are reminded that medicine is a constantly evolving science and while the authors and publishers have ensured that all dosages, applications and practices are based on current indications, there may be specific practices which differ between communities. You should always follow the guidelines laid down by the manufacturers of specific products and the relevant authorities in the country in which you are practising.

Although every effort has been made to ensure that all owners of copyright material have been acknowledged in this publication, we would be pleased to acknowledge in subsequent reprints or editions any omissions brought to our attention.

Registered names, trademarks, etc. used in this book, even when not marked as such, are not to be considered unprotected by law.

Use the free Learning Diary app from FourteenFish to record your notes and reflection as you read this book.

www.fourteenfish.com/app

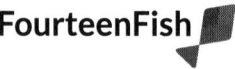

Cover design by Andrew Magee Design Ltd.

Typeset by Evolution Design & Digital Ltd (Kent)

Printed in the UK

Last digit is the print number: 10 9 8 7 6 5 4 3 2

Contents

Preface   *vii*

Acknowledgements   *viii*

Contributors   *viii*

Dedications   *viii*

Abbreviations   *ix*

How to use this book   *xi*

Chapter 1 Ask the allergist   **1**
  1.1   What is an allergy?   2
  1.2   What is an allergic reaction?   2
  1.3   What are common types of allergens?   2
  1.4   Where does the immune system come into this?   6
  1.5   What is hypersensitivity?   11
  1.6   How big a problem is allergy?   17
  1.7   What is new in allergy treatment?   17

Chapter 2 Clinical assessment of the allergic patient   **19**
  2.1   History-taking in allergy   20
  2.2   Clinical examination in the allergic patient   22
  2.3   Investigations   22
  2.4   Radiological imaging   31

Chapter 3 Clinical allergy   **33**
  3.1   Systemic allergy   34
  3.2   Skin allergies   39
  3.3   Eye   41
  3.4   Nose and sinus   42

3.5	Ear	44
3.6	Respiratory	44
3.7	Food and oral allergies	46
3.8	Drug allergy	50
3.9	Latex allergy	51
3.10	Insect allergy	51
3.11	Others	52

Chapter 4 Asthma: background and clinical presentation **55**
4.1	Pathophysiology	56
4.2	Risk factors for asthma	57
4.3	Stratification of asthma	57
4.4	Diagnosis	57
4.5	Differential diagnoses	60
4.6	Asthma attack	63
4.7	Complications of asthma	63

Chapter 5 Asthma: management **65**
5.1	Acute asthma management	66
5.2	Chronic asthma management	67
5.3	Monitoring asthma	73
5.4	Paediatric asthma	74

Chapter 6 Management principles in allergy **77**
6.1	Pharmacotherapy	78

Chapter 7 Organ-specific treatment **85**
7.1	Skin	86
7.2	Nose and sinuses	86
7.3	Ear	88
7.4	Eye	89
7.5	Chest and abdomen	89

Chapter 8 Allergy in children **91**
8.1	Clinical assessment of allergy in children	93
8.2	Investigating allergy in children	94
8.3	Food allergy	95
8.4	Asthma	95

Index *97*

Preface

Allergic diseases are common; in fact, they are the most common chronic condition in Europe. It is estimated that a fifth of patients with allergies struggle every day with the fear of a possible asthma attack, anaphylactic shock or even death from an allergic reaction. A book like this, a complete go-to resource for clinicians managing allergy, is therefore much needed.

This book is a guide for those in primary care, for hospital doctors including trainees, for medical students, and for specialist healthcare workers including specialist nurses interested in the rapidly expanding field of allergy. It covers the range of common and important conditions, outlining good clinical practice. You are taken from the basic science through diagnosis, investigations and management. For primary care, support for the decision-making process to onward referral to specialist services is also provided.

The book begins by systematically covering the basics and then walks you through diagnosis of key conditions and how to manage them in detail, including the latest asthma guidelines. Diagnosis of allergy is crucial, as it often presents as complex syndromes. It requires a comprehensive yet clinically applicable understanding of the immune system and its role in homeostasis. The patient must be carefully assessed and given a targeted management plan. All have been described here in a complete and easy-to-understand narrative. The book also covers the pressing issue of paediatric allergy; labelling a child with 'asthma' or as an 'allergy sufferer' implies potentially lifelong specialist care, social environmental care and NHS funding.

The author has in-depth knowledge of the subject and long experience of managing allergic patients, in both adult and paediatric specialist services.

The principles shown here represent a handy blend of expertise and evidence-based recommendations to allow you to manage your patients with confidence and with good outcomes.

Dr Amtul Salam Sami

Acknowledgements

I am very grateful to my children and my husband; the time they gave, their support and their inspiration are deeply valued.

Contributors

Thank you to Dr Nida Ahmed and Mr Sabahat Ahmed for their hard work and consistent commitment.

Dedications

I dedicate this book to my parents, Dr Abdul Sami and Amtul Rehman Sami.

Abbreviations

ABCDE	airway, breathing, circulation, disability and exposure
ACE	angiotensin-converting enzyme
BTS	British Thoracic Society
CT	computed tomography
DPI	dry powder inhaler
ELISA	enzyme-linked immunosorbent assay
ENT	ear, nose and throat
FeNO	fraction exhaled nitric oxide
FEV_1	forced expiratory volume in 1 second
FVC	forced vital capacity
HDM	house dust mite
HLA	human leukocyte antigen
ICS	inhaled corticosteroid
IM	intramuscular
ITU	intensive therapy unit
IV	intravenous
LABA	long-acting beta-2 agonist
LTRA	leukotriene receptor antagonist
MART	maintenance and reliever therapy

MBL   mannose-binding lectin

MDI   metered-dose inhaler

MHC   major histocompatibility complex

NICE   National Institute for Health and Care Excellence

NK   natural killer

NSAID   non-steroidal anti-inflammatory drug

OAS   oral allergy syndrome

PFS   pollen fruit syndrome

PND   paroxysmal nocturnal dyspnoea

ppb   parts per billion

RAST   radioallergosorbent test

SABA   short-acting beta-2 agonist

SIGN   Scottish Intercollegiate Guideline Network

SLE   systemic lupus erythematosus

How to use this book

A working understanding of the immune system including its components and the pathophysiology behind allergic disease is key to recognising its wide-reaching implications. The basics you need have been laid out at the beginning of this book, in *Chapter 1, Ask the allergist*. Use this to provide you with a sturdy foundation before diving into the various clinical presentations and relating them to the patients you see.

Chapter 1
Ask the allergist

1.1	What is an allergy?	2
1.2	What is an allergic reaction?	2
1.3	What are common types of allergens?	2
1.4	Where does the immune system come into this?	6
1.5	What is hypersensitivity?	11
1.6	How big a problem is allergy?	17
1.7	What is new in allergy treatment?	17

This chapter provides the key basic principles needed to understand allergy as seen clinically. Assessment of the allergic patient, diagnosis of individual conditions and management are covered in their own chapters later in the book.

1.1 What is an allergy?

Simply put, an allergy represents malfunction of the immune system when it is exposed to an otherwise harmless allergen.

An allergen is an antigen that can trigger an allergy. An antigen is the basic element capable of initiating an immune response in a host with sensitised antibodies or lymphocytes. Allergens can be proteins, glycoproteins, carbohydrates or even abnormal complexes formed by chemical modification of the host's own proteins.

An allergic reaction involves various cells and mediators. Allergic disorders have characteristic features depending on whether the allergen is inhaled, ingested, injected or otherwise contacted. Atopic individuals are those prone to developing an allergy.

1.2 What is an allergic reaction?

An allergic reaction is the symptomatology that develops as a result of the allergic response; the response is the pathogenesis when the immune system is triggered to defensive action against an allergen. It can affect many body systems (see the clinical allergy section, in which each one is covered separately). Severity can vary: at worst, an allergic reaction can be life-threatening.

1.3 What are common types of allergens?

Allergens are diverse in nature and are harmless to the non-allergic individual. Allergens to which humans are often exposed include:
- airborne allergens, e.g. house dust mite, grass pollen (especially timothy grass), weed pollen (ragweed in particular) and tree pollen (especially birch)
- insect bites/stings, animal dander, animal secretions, moulds such as *Alternaria*, *Cladosporium*, *Aspergillus*, *Penicillium* and *Fusarium* species
- food allergens, commonly including eggs, milk, nuts (and peanuts, although technically these are legumes), seafood (including shellfish), soybeans, wheat and some types of fruit
- occupational allergens, including flour, wood, cotton, various plastics and chemical compounds
- miscellaneous, including some drugs, metals, rubber, nylon and latex.

Sensitivity to one allergen can sometimes imply sensitivity to related substances. For example, people with an allergy to penicillin can have a high level of cross-reactivity with carbapenems; those with latex allergy can have cross-reactivity with foodstuffs including bananas, avocados and kiwi fruit, amongst others; individuals sensitive to house dust mites may also react to wheat and some seafoods, such as lobster.

Let's look at some common allergens in more detail (see also *Figure 1.1*).

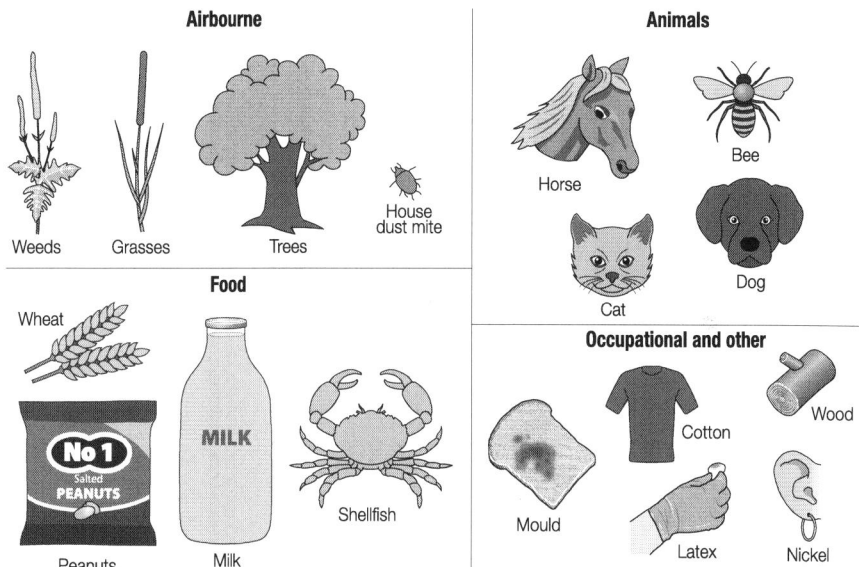

Figure 1.1 Common allergens.

1.3.1 Fungi as allergens

Moulds are a form of fungus. There are thousands of species of mould in the UK, present all year round both indoors and outdoors. They are found on plants in the garden, on farms, in food stores (including cupboards) and homes. Outdoors, the level of moulds in the air usually reaches its peak in the evening hours. They have a strong affinity to damp, with decaying vegetation promoting heavy mould growth. Indoors, moulds grow anywhere where moisture collects: beneath and around drains, in basements, garages, near water leaks and drips, even around indoor plants and bird droppings in bird cages.

The symptoms of patients with a mould allergy often get worse in autumn and winter. In order to limit the growth of moulds, the home should have an adequate level of dry heating. Ventilation should be sufficient to prevent vapour from cooking, boiling water or drying clothes on radiators from accumulating and increasing humidity. Other measures include ensuring that storage cupboards are not overfilled, as that can affect the ventilation of the area. Existing moulds can be cleaned away with bleach or commercial chemicals specifically made to remove them. Where mould growth is not under control, professional help should be sought from building research advisory services. Remember, treating the mould source(s) may eliminate the patient's problem altogether.

1.3.2 House dust and house dust mites as allergens

House dust is made up of a combination of many substances including toxic chemical compounds found in some aerosols, clothing fibres, sloughed skin, bacteria and house dust mites (HDMs). HDMs are microscopic, spider-like organisms found in fabric, upholstery, bed linen, pillows, mattresses and carpets; they live on the dead skin cells that are shed from human bodies every day. The major allergen from HDMs is an aggressive digestive enzyme found in the droppings, which can affect the lining of the upper airway including nose, sinuses, lungs and eyes. The worst allergy season for HDM-sensitive individuals is winter, when closed, warm, cosy houses create a favourable environment for HDMs.

Allergic individuals should use more than one method of clearing HDMs; removing carpets decreases the reservoir of HDMs, as does washing fluffy toys, and washing bedding (with a preference for cotton as opposed to synthetic materials) at higher temperatures to kill HDMs and remove allergens. Lowering indoor humidity by air conditioning or central heating, according to the weather, also controls HDM growth. Vacuuming carpets at least once a week will remove faecal pellets in dust, but not live HDMs. Allergen-proof covers for pillowcases and mattresses significantly improve patients' symptoms. There is a lot of information available online about HDM avoidance, and about cleaning products and gadgets to help remove them. Nevertheless, unfortunately, a significant number of patients need to use treatment (albeit only a minimal therapy burden), either in the form of nasal sprays or inhalers, which may be required only in the winter.

1.3.3 Animal allergens

Another common form of allergy in atopic individuals is caused by the airborne secretions, fur or feathers of pets such as cats, dogs, rabbits, horses or birds, or rodents or insects such as cockroaches.

The release of allergens from household pets occurs when the pet licks its fur; the allergens in the saliva dry and fall when the hair falls. These allergens coat the area where they fall (for example a carpet, bedding or clothes). Cat and dog allergens can also be found in schools and community areas in sufficient quantity to initiate allergic symptoms in atopic individuals.

The major cat allergen is the protein Fel d 1. The particles are typically 2.5 microns in diameter and remain airborne for long enough in quantities sufficient to provoke symptoms. These allergens adhere to carpets, drapes, bedding and clothing, and can be detected for up to 16 weeks, or sometimes even longer, after removal of the cat from a house. Dog, rabbit, horse and rodent allergens are less persistent, but they can provoke symptoms of similar severity. In some cases, people living with a pet may not notice any symptoms but when they stay away for a few weeks and then return they may notice the symptoms of allergy.

The best treatment is to find the pet a new home, then clean the house thoroughly including the carpet, linen and walls of the rooms where the pet spent most time. However, the emotional and psychological consequences for the individual of removing the pet can be significant. Alternatively, it may be an idea not to replace the pet when it dies. If it is not possible to remove the pet, then the patient's bedroom should become a pet-free area, the pet should be washed at least once a week, and the pet's sitting area should be thoroughly cleaned at least twice a week.

If symptomatic, the atopic individual should use medication as advised. In severe cases immunotherapy can be advised in specialist centres under allergy specialist assessment and management.

1.3.4 Grass and tree pollen as allergens

Grass pollen and tree pollen are responsible for seasonal symptoms from allergic rhinitis to seasonal asthma. In the case of tree pollen, symptoms usually start around the end of February, whilst grass pollen season is around May to July.

There are simple avoidance measures which can help to minimise the symptoms and improve quality of life, such as:
- avoiding areas of recently cut grass
- avoiding gardening or (if it is necessary) taking a shower including washing the hair thoroughly immediately afterwards
- keeping house and car windows shut in the pollen season and, where possible, using the car air filter or air conditioning
- using a light coating of petroleum jelly around the outer rim of the nostrils (simply applied with a fingertip).

If medication has been prescribed, then it should be used in addition to allergen avoidance.

If the patient is unresponsive to treatment and no issues with technique or concordance are identified, or if their symptoms are affecting their quality of life, then they should be referred to an allergist for further expert advice and consideration for immunotherapy.

1.4 Where does the immune system come into this?

The immune system's basic function is to protect the body from harmful stimuli. There are physical barriers that stop allergens and microbes from entering the body (see *Figure 1.2*). The immune system also has a variety of cells and mediators present in the circulatory system and in tissues that work individually or in collaboration with each other to identify and neutralise harmful substances to which the body is exposed, through immune-mediated inflammation and influencing activation of immune cells.

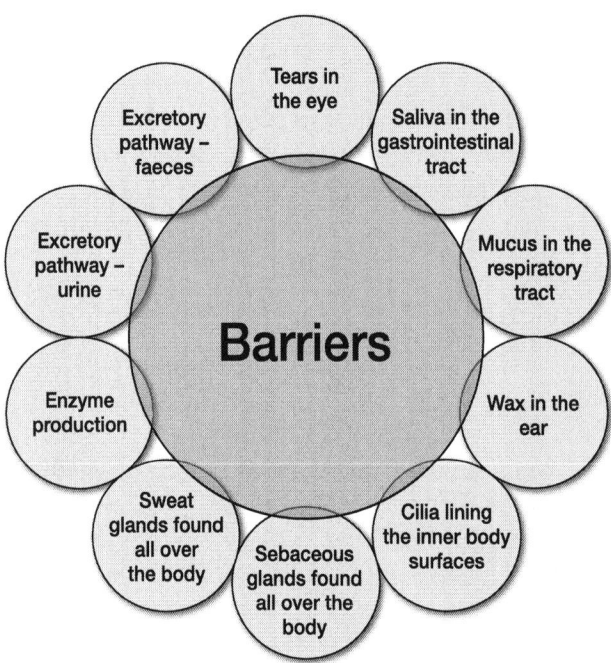

Figure 1.2 Natural barriers present in the defence of the human body.

The immune system can correctly function only when self/non-self stimuli and harmful/non-harmful stimuli are appropriately differentiated. In autoimmune diseases the former fails, whereas in allergy, the latter fails. Allergic diseases are complex disorders, resulting from a combination of factors including genetic tendency, environmental factors (including air pollution) and *in utero* exposures, such as smoking and some drugs. Various studies on the timing of action of genetic variants in determining disease susceptibility have highlighted the importance of *in utero* development and early life upbringing in determining allergic disease.

The immune system has an innate response (an inborn but limited system, see below) and an adaptive response (a slower and more specific process).

1.4.1 Innate immunity

Innate immunity is the first-line defence the immune system offers. It relies on pattern recognition based on a relatively small collection of receptors that are non-specific in nature (because the receptors are inherited through the genome, they do not require any previous exposure to pathogens to form). Its key components are listed in *Table 1.1*. This system is also involved in readying the adaptive immune system (see later) and has a role in defence against tumours.

Table 1.1 Key components of the innate immune system.

Cells	Soluble mediators
Monocytes	Complement
Macrophages	Defensins
Dendritic cells	Cytokines
Neutrophils	
Eosinophils	
Basophils	
Natural killer cells	
Natural killer T cells	

Going into the stimulating details of the innate immune system digresses from the focus of this book, but there are a few key facts about this remarkable system that are helpful to know. It is fast-acting (minutes to hours) and is fundamentally based on self/non-self discrimination. It does not provide long-lasting immunity to the host.

When activated, the innate immune system stimulates the complement cascade (see below) leading to the destruction of offending organisms by the cells and mediators listed in *Table 1.1*. Of note, natural killer (NK) cells also have the capacity to rapidly kill malignant cells.

1.4.2 The complement system

Complement plays a critical role in inflammation and defence against bodily insult, and it can contribute to both innate and adaptive immune responses. It comprises over twenty proteins (synthesised in the liver), which act as the initial point in a biochemical cascade that helps the body to clear pathogens or prepare them for destruction by other cells. These proteins are found circulating in blood and in tissues and are activated by one of the three pathways (classical, alternative or lectin; see *Figure 1.3*).

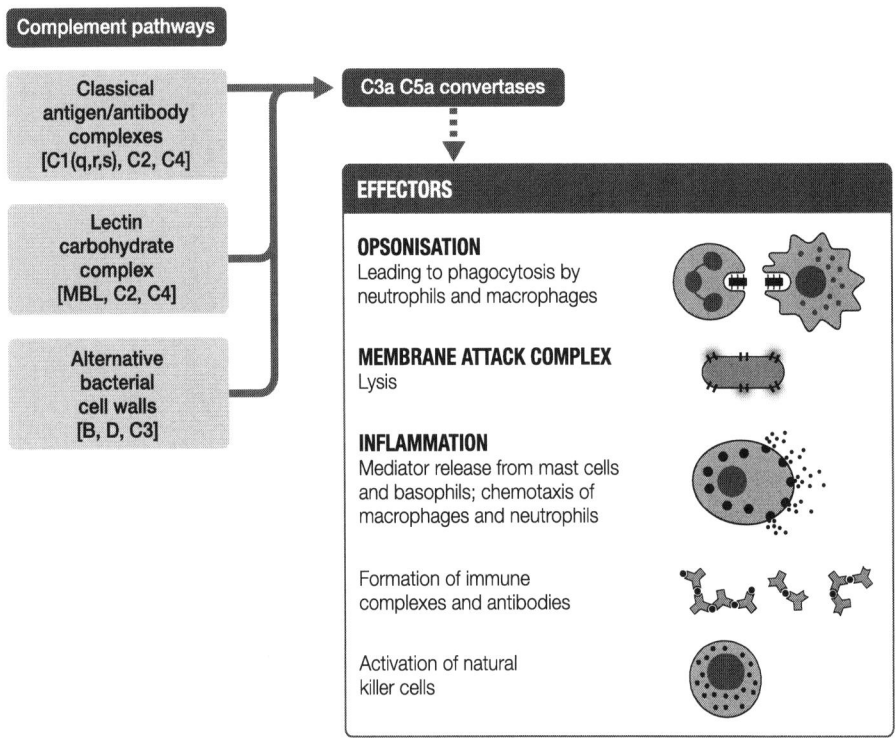

Figure 1.3 Simplified complement cascade. The dashed line indicates that there are many steps between these two processes. B, Factor B; C refers to the many proteins found in the complement cascade; D, Factor D; MBL, mannose-binding lectin.
Adapted from *Anatomy and Physiology in Healthcare* by Marshall *et al.* (2017), © Scion Publishing Ltd.

The classical pathway is activated via the antigen–antibody complex (see *Section 1.4.4*). The alternative pathway is stimulated by the innate immune system (see above), that is, it is not triggered by an antibody or the specific structure of a pathogen, and it is in a constant state of activation; it can proceed on any microbial surface or abnormal host tissue. The lectin pathway is mediated by the binding of mannose-binding lectin, which recognises and binds to specific sugars that are typically found only on foreign bodies.

All of these pathways involve complement component C3, which, through the action of C3 convertase, is divided into long and small segments; C3b is a long segment that acts as an opsonin (a powerful promotor of phagocytosis), whilst the small segment C3a promotes inflammation and triggers the destruction of pathogens by activation of phagocytic cells.

There are diseases attributed to complement deficiencies or abnormal functioning of complement, with continued research being carried out in this arena. Those individuals who lack one of the proteins of the membrane attack complex (C5b, C6, C7, C8 and C9 form a complex that ultimately induces cell lysis; *Figure 1.3*) can be predisposed to *Neisseria meningitidis*; deficiency in C1, C4 or C2 can predispose to systemic lupus erythematosus (SLE) and glomerulonephritis; C1 inhibitor deficiency can predispose to angioedema.

1.4.3 Adaptive immunity

The adaptive immune response is antigen-specific (it recognises unique structural features of the index pathogen) and includes immunological memory, so can produce targeted antibodies on second or repeated exposure to the same pathogen. It is, however, slower than the innate system, which simply relies on pattern recognition.

The key cells involved in the adaptive immune system are B lymphocytes (B cells) and T lymphocytes (T cells). T cells are further split into helper (CD4) T cells, cytotoxic (CD8) T cells and regulatory T cells; the last are important in the elimination of T cells that recognise self-antigens. B cells mediate humoral immunity; they secrete antibodies into extracellular fluids. T cells mediate cell-mediated immunity; specific cytotoxic T cells are produced and support for the activity of phagocytic cells is intensified.

1.4.4 Lymphocytes

The lymphocytes of the adaptive immune system deserve special attention given that they are key components of allergic disorders.

After production and early development in the bone marrow, B cells move to the lymphatic system to mature. Each B cell has on its surface an antigen-specific B-cell receptor (derived from the host's genetic make-up). The B-cell receptor is a membrane-bound form of the antibody that it will later secrete. When an antigen matches this receptor, it activates a pathway dividing the B cell (at this point termed a naive B cell) to form memory B cells and plasma cells.

Memory B cells express the same membrane-bound immunoglobulin on their surface as the original naive B cell. Plasma B cells secrete free immunoglobulins as antibodies (see *Section 1.4.5*) which then bind to the antigen. In the initial stage, the secreted antibody is an immunoglobulin type M; the B cells later 'switch' to the production of immunoglobulin type G. The antibody–antigen complex activates the complement cascade via activation of the classical pathway (see *Section 1.4.2*), leading to termination of the pathogen, either directly or through activation of phagocytosis.

B cells also release cytokines, with an immunoregulatory role, and function as antigen-presenting cells for presentation to T helper cells.

T cells are formed in the bone marrow and migrate to the thymus gland to mature. In the thymus, T cells undergo two selection processes: positive selection (elimination of those T cells that fail to interact with host major histocompatibility complex, MHC) and negative selection (elimination of those T cells that recognise self peptides).

T cells express T-cell receptors, which recognise antigens bound to MHC (membrane-bound surface receptors on antigen-presenting cells). The function of the MHC is to bind antigens from pathogens and present them on the cell surface for recognition by the appropriate T cells.

There are three types of mature T cells:
- T helper cells: These express CD4 receptors and aid activation of key immune cells, including B cells, cytotoxic T cells, dendritic cells and macrophages, through release of cytokines. These cells subsequently mature into either type 1 (Th1), which are important against intracellular pathogens and mycobacteria, or type 2 (Th2), which produce a group of cytokines involved in B-cell immunoglobulin switching, including IgE production (see *Section 1.4.5*). It is known that people with a high Th1:Th2 ratio are less likely to develop allergy, while those with a low Th1:Th2 ratio are much more likely to develop allergy and asthma.
- Cytotoxic T cells: These express CD8 receptors and play a crucial role in the control of intracellular pathogens. They can kill cells through inducing lysis or apoptosis, or secrete cytokines that are pro-inflammatory or will attract more lymphocytes to the area.
- T regulatory cells: These express CD4 and CD25 receptors, help to distinguish between self and non-self and help prevent autoimmune diseases.

1.4.5 Antibodies

Antibodies are present in extracellular fluids (humoral immunity; see *Section 1.4.4*). An antibody is a Y-shaped immunoglobulin protein (*Figure 1.4*) produced mainly by plasma B cells in response to a specific antigen, whether free or on the surface of the pathogens. It binds directly to these antigens. Antibodies can be one of five classes, IgA, IgD, IgE, IgG and IgM, the name denoting the varying heavy chains in each distinct class. IgE in particular has an integral role in the development of allergy.

The ultimate function of an antibody is to neutralise pathogens such as bacteria and viruses. There is a binding site for the respective antigen on each tip of the Y segment of the antibody. The antibody communicates with components of the immune system via the Fc receptor region.

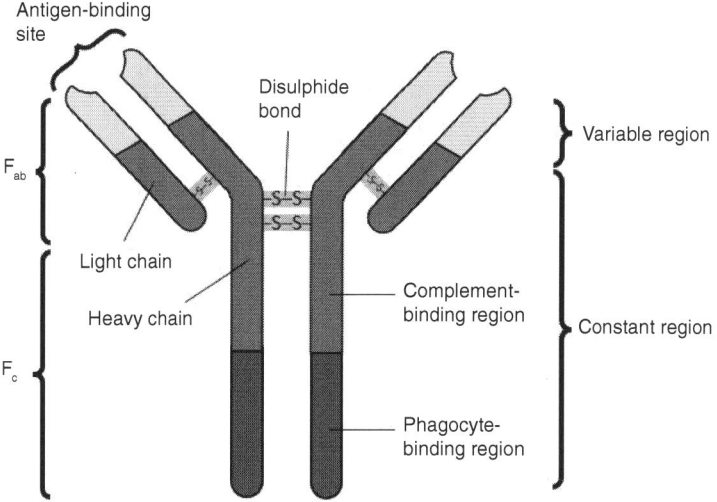

Figure 1.4 Basic structure of an immunoglobulin.

1.5 What is hypersensitivity?

Immunologically, allergy can be split into four types of reaction, defined by (and named after) R Coombs and PGH Gell in 1968; these are summarised in *Table 1.2*.

Table 1.2 Summary of Gell–Coombs classification of hypersensitivity reactions.

Reaction type	Mechanism
I	Anaphylactic, IgE-dependent
II	Cytotoxic
III	Damage by toxic complexes
IV	Delayed, cell-mediated

1.5.1 Type I reaction

The type I hypersensitivity reaction is represented in *Figure 1.5*. The allergen can enter the body through various routes, for example respiratory, gastrointestinal (in food or medications), insect stings or physical contact. The allergen is then phagocytosed by macrophages, to be processed and positioned on their surface for presentation to receptors on T helper cells. Cell-to-cell contact with naive B cells leads to their activation, producing plasma cells capable of producing allergen-specific antibodies.

In allergic patients, these plasma cells produce large amounts of allergen-specific IgE, under the control of cytokines and mediators, which binds to mast cells

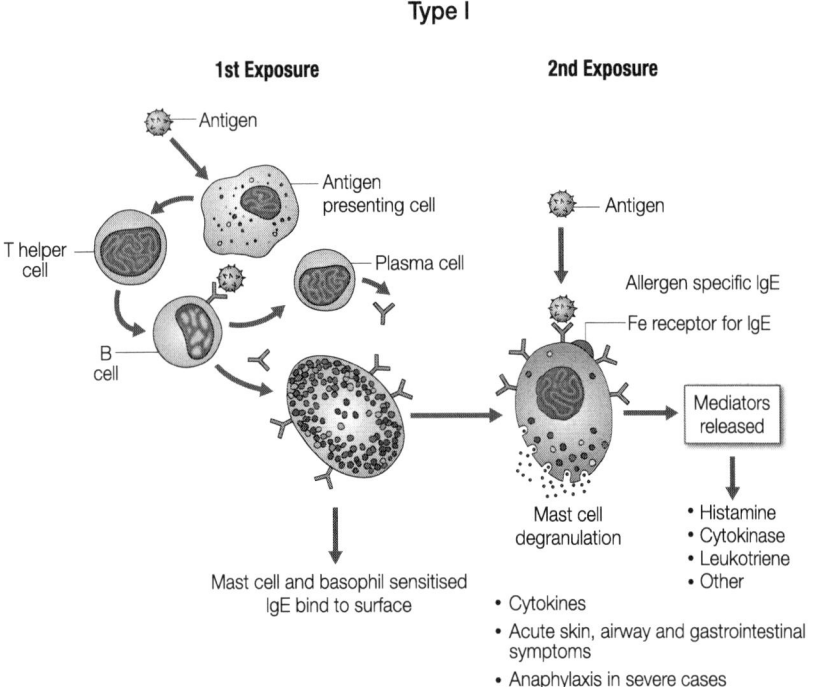

Figure 1.5 Type I hypersensitivity reaction: the reaction begins with first exposure and subsequent sensitisation to the allergen. The next exposure to that allergen or its metabolite leads to an IgE-mediated allergic reaction.

throughout the body. Mast cells and basophils contain granules that contain histamine and various chemical mediators. Histamine, once released into tissues or the bloodstream, binds to histamine receptors on blood vessels, mucous glands and the respiratory tract, causing some of the typical symptoms seen in an allergic reaction such as cough and shortness of breath.

The type I reaction has an early phase and a late phase. The main mediators of the early phase are histamine (as above) and prostaglandin D2 (a very potent contributor to inflammation in the respiratory tract). They act as vasodilators in the systemic circulation and cause bronchoconstriction (producing wheeze, oedema and increased mucous secretions) as well as the classical urticarial rash.

The late phase is due to mediators that are simultaneously released by the mast cells at the time of degranulation. These signal the influx of other inflammatory cells, including T cells and other granulocytes (e.g. neutrophils and eosinophils), which initiate an inflammatory reaction of lower intensity but longer duration. Indeed, some chemical mediators are not formed until 5–30 minutes after activation of mast cells or basophils. Mediators of the late-phase response are interleukin-4 and 5 (responsible for leukocyte activation), tumour necrosis factor-alpha, leukotriene C4 (which increases endothelial cell adhesion), eosinophil chemotactic factor (responsible for leukocyte migration) and platelet-activating factor.

Another major mediator of the type I reaction is the leukotriene D4, which is significantly more potent than histamine and can also attract other immune cells to aggravate the inflammation. Other mediators include thromboxane, cytokines, free radicals, kinins and adenosine.

After the resolution of the inflammatory response, a population of lymphocytes remains in the circulation and peripheral tissue as memory cells able to identify the allergen and initiate the entire sequence of events again. Therefore, patients remain susceptible to a reaction upon re-exposure for many years or even for their lifetime. An important point to note is that this is the only type of allergic reaction that can be diagnosed reliably by skin-prick test and also by *in vitro* testing.

Clinically, this reaction type can present as allergic rhinitis, asthma and anaphylaxis. Anaphylaxis represents the most severe form. It is an immediate reaction, occurring in a matter of seconds or minutes, and can be lethal.

1.5.2 Type II reaction

In a type II reaction, antibodies cause immune-mediated cell destruction (*Figure 1.6*). Antibodies (commonly IgG or, less frequently, IgM) target antigens on the surface of the foreign cell, or membrane-bound antigens. The consequent reaction, mediated either by complement or by cytotoxic T cells, causes cell damage including cell lysis.

Clinically, conditions attributed to this reaction include Graves' disease, myasthenia gravis and haemolytic disease of the newborn. Graves' disease is a form of hyperthyroidism, the basis of which is the formation of anti-receptor antibodies (antibodies against the thyroid-stimulating hormone receptor) which interrupt the normal thyroid homeostasis mechanism. In myasthenia gravis, acetylcholine receptor antibodies impair neuromuscular transmission. In haemolytic disease of the newborn, the blood of the Rhesus-positive foetus leaks across the blood–placenta barrier into the Rhesus-negative mother, who forms anti-Rhesus antibodies. In subsequent pregnancies with a Rhesus-positive foetus, foetal red blood cells are destroyed, with potentially fatal complications.

Other diseases involving a type II hypersensitivity reaction are:
- bullous pemphigoid
- cytopenia – thrombocytopenia, agranulocytosis

Type II

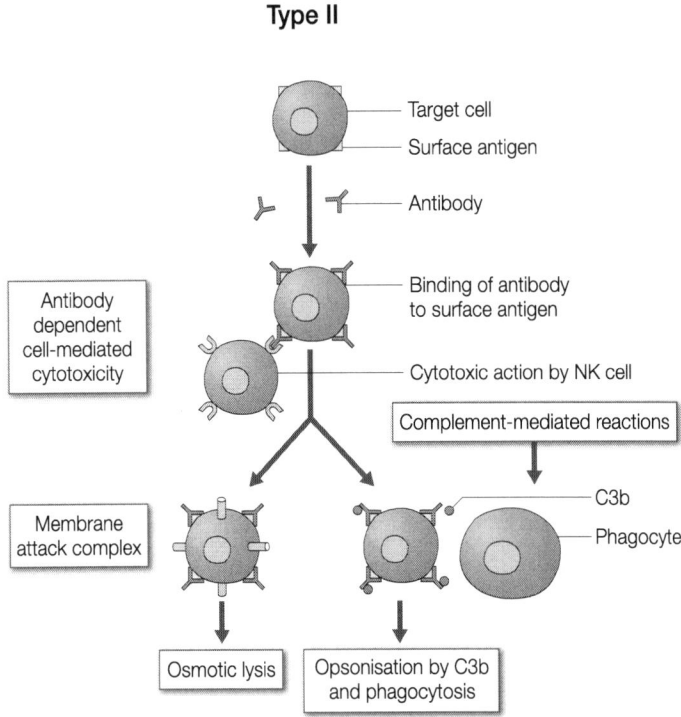

Figure 1.6 Type II hypersensitivity reaction: the specific antibody binds to its target, starting a process that results in cell death either by the cytotoxic action of NK cells or via complement, through membrane attack complex or phagocytosis.

- haemolytic anaemia in some drug allergies, e.g. penicillin
- Goodpasture's syndrome
- hyperacute graft rejection.

Instead of binding to cell surfaces, the antibodies recognise and bind to the cell surface receptors, either preventing the intended ligand from binding with the receptor or mimicking the effects of the ligand, thus impairing cell signalling.

1.5.3 Type III reaction

Antibody–antigen complexes form an immune complex in a type III reaction (*Figure 1.7*). An antigen enters the body and reacts with circulating antibodies (IgM and IgG) to form irregular molecular aggregates called immune complexes. Normally these immune complexes are cleared from the body promptly by the reticuloendothelial system; however, in type III reactions this is not the case,

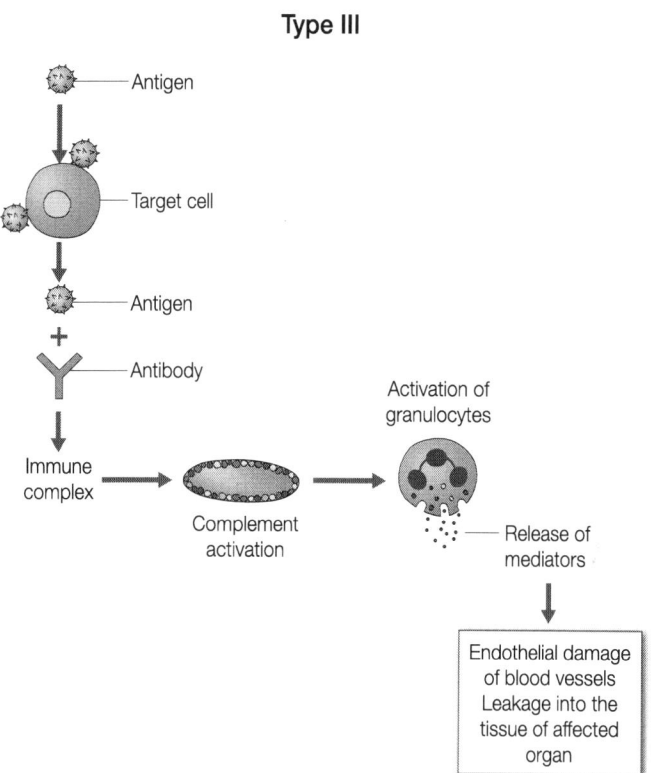

Figure 1.7 Type III hypersensitivity reaction: when the antibody combines with its specific antigen, immune complexes are formed. Wherever immune complexes are deposited, they activate the complement system, and macrophages and neutrophils are attracted to the site, where they cause inflammation leading to tissue injury.

so they are deposited in host tissues, causing damage. Circulating immune complexes start depositing along the small vessels of various target organs, precipitating an inflammatory reaction attracting cellular debris (in the form of basophils, polymorphs, leukocytes and platelets). This results in the release of mediators that cause retraction of the endothelial cells lining the small blood vessels of the target organ. Hence fluid and inflammatory substances can leak into the tissue.

The reaction can take hours or days (even weeks in some cases), depending in part on the presence of immunological memory of the precipitating antigen. The response can also become chronic, particularly in autoimmune reactions, where antigen persists. Clinical examples of type III reactions are glomerulonephritis, vasculitis, rheumatoid arthritis and SLE.

1.5.4 Type IV reaction

A type IV hypersensitivity reaction involves T-cell-mediated cell death (*Figure 1.8*), known as a 'delayed-type' reaction owing to the time taken to activate T cells. This delayed reaction (generally occurring 24–48 hours after contact, even up to 72 hours) is mediated by T cells activated after the allergen was processed and exposed on the antigen-presenting cells' surface MHC molecules. The Th1 cells secrete cytokines that activate macrophages and cytotoxic T cells.

Clinically, examples of type IV reactions include contact dermatitis, tuberculin skin reaction, Hashimoto's thyroiditis, primary biliary cholangitis, chronic asthma and chronic allergic rhinitis. A common routine example is the delayed skin reaction produced after contact with poison ivy.

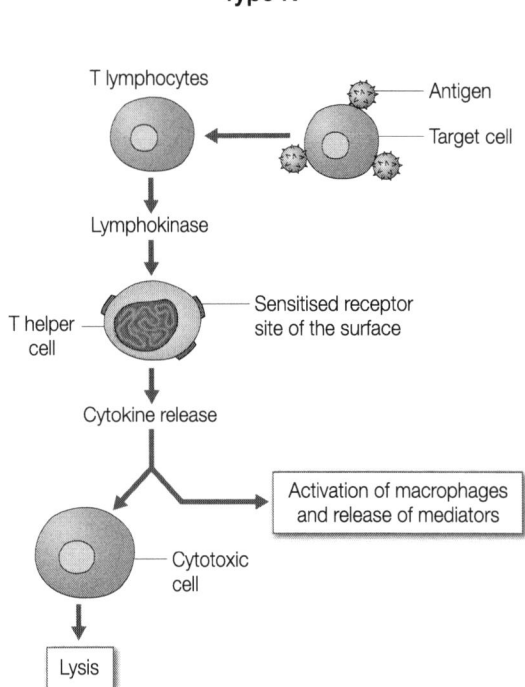

Figure 1.8 Type IV hypersensitivity reaction: the antigen is processed and presented on an antigen-presenting cell. T-cell receptors interact with this exposed antigen, thus triggering inflammation and ultimately destruction by the cytotoxic T cell.

1.5.5 Fixed and cyclic types

As well as the immunological classification of allergies by Gell–Coombs reaction types, a clinical classification into fixed and cyclic allergy types is also recognised (mainly in the USA, less so in the UK).

A fixed allergy is an IgE-mediated response and manifests as an immediate reaction (within seconds, up to a few hours) after contact with allergens to which the individual is sensitised. Most drug allergies, insect sting allergy and some food allergies are of this type. Even after a period of no contact with the allergen, re-exposure will usually fully re-establish the reaction. Clinically it should be considered a permanent allergy and the offending allergen should be avoided.

Cyclic allergy is both dose- and frequency-related and is not IgE-mediated. The reaction is delayed (range: <1 hour to a couple of days). Food sensitivities are usually of this type; however, this is not exclusively the case, for example the seasonal priming effect of inhaled allergens. At the start of allergy season the patient may have mild symptoms, but as the season progresses, the allergy becomes more severe as the entire immune system becomes progressively more sensitive. After the priming effect, repeated exposure (even to a small amount which earlier caused only mild symptoms) evokes a more symptomatic response with more rapid onset.

1.6 How big a problem is allergy?

Allergy is the most common chronic disease in Europe and has a rising incidence; according to the World Allergy Organization, more than 150 million Europeans have chronic allergic diseases. The current prediction is that by 2025 half of the entire population of Europe will be affected; the UK has some of the highest prevalences of allergic conditions worldwide.

1.7 What is new in allergy treatment?

Whilst human leukocyte antigen (HLA) associations have been identified, as well as gene associations with interleukins, ADAM33 metalloproteinase and high-affinity IgE receptor beta-subunit, research is still active in this area. Ongoing scientific research continues to clarify the mechanisms involved in allergic reactions, pointing towards more effective treatment and allergy prevention. Indeed, there is hope that vaccines for certain allergies will be available in future.

Effective therapies for allergies, such as immunotherapies, are increasingly used. They aim to minimise the reaction itself rather than to target the symptoms. Research is also being done into prevention of allergy through factors related to lifestyle, upbringing and food, which may affect guidelines in the future.

Chapter 2

Clinical assessment of the allergic patient

2.1   History-taking in allergy   20

2.2   Clinical examination in the allergic patient   22

2.3   Investigations   22

2.4   Radiological imaging   31

Allergy can present in a variety of ways. It can be an acute or a chronic issue and often presents with signs and symptoms that occur in non-allergic conditions as well. Clinical examples of this observation:

- repeated ear infections or serous otitis media in children may have an allergic cause, rather than being related to Eustachian tube anatomy
- a patient with unexplained rash and lethargy could have an allergic aetiology
- a migraine-type headache or gastrointestinal symptoms could be allergic in nature
- feeling unwell after eating sugary food may not have an endocrine basis but rather an allergic cause
- a red eye does not always mean infection; it could be an allergy.

Diagnosing allergy requires a good, detailed history (most important part of making the diagnosis), clinical examination and the appropriate investigations (the tests required depend on the type of allergen being investigated). These are all covered in detail under the relevant headings.

It is important that patients with a suspected allergy, even if it is clinically evident at first presentation, should be referred to an allergy clinic with the advice to avoid the suspected allergen until review. If the allergy is anaphylactic they should also be provided with an adrenaline auto-injector. Allergy services can provide specialist tests (including checking for cross-reactivity) and treatments under supervision that may not be available to patients not seen by a specialist.

2.1 History-taking in allergy

This section focuses on aspects of the history pertinent to allergic disease. However, it is still necessary to take a comprehensive history (see *Figure 2.1* for the basic layout). Each positive symptom will need to be explored and the presence of associated symptoms reviewed. It is of paramount importance to explore the patient's ideas, concerns and expectations.

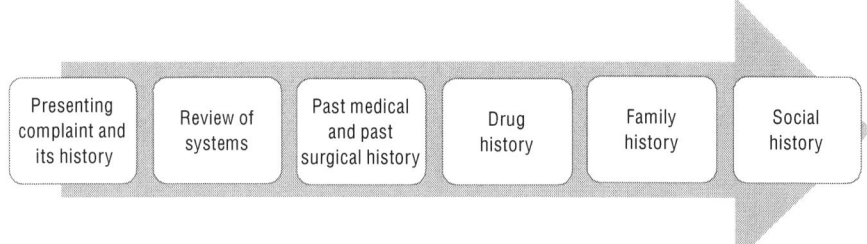

Figure 2.1 Scheme for taking a comprehensive history.

Allergy can present as a complex entity with great variation between patients; in severe cases the patient may be unconscious, in which case the collateral history will be of upmost importance.

As there are many different types of allergy with different routes of exposure (including inhalant, ingestion and direct skin contact) it can present with symptoms affecting different organs, as listed in *Figure 2.2*; this provides a clear history framework which can be applied to help screen for multiple pathologies that may be caused by an allergen(s).

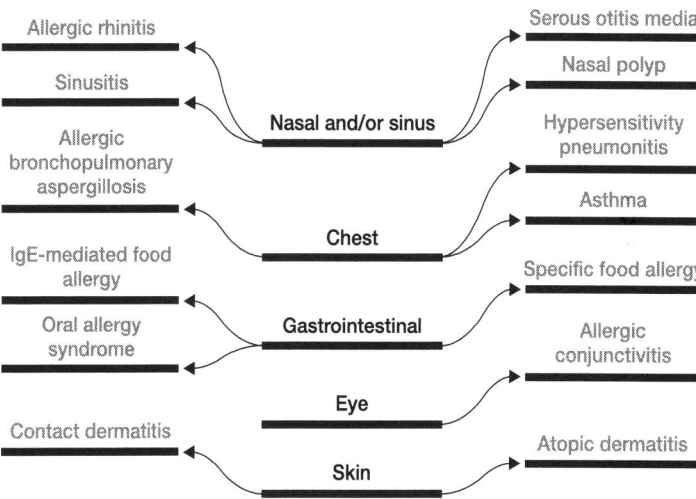

Figure 2.2 List of organ systems and the associated diseases that should be screened for when assessing the allergic patient.

In every history, questions should cover the index event (if acute) and its temporal relationship to the symptoms (including severity). If an occupational allergen is suspected, check for any change in the patient's symptomatology when they go on holiday.

When the lesion is on the skin then location may indicate the causative agent. Look for locations where fashion accessories or jewellery are worn (body piercings, wrists, neck etc.), or if the lesion is on the face check cosmetics use. Remember also to screen for associated symptoms of other common allergic conditions.

With allergy, there are additional avenues to explore depending on the progress of the history. Be sure to ask about reactions to insect bites. In the case of environmental or occupational allergy, for example latex allergy in individuals working in the cleaning industry or hay fever in gardeners, questions regarding housing, hobbies and occupation (including workplace) are important.

Medication history, including allergies to any medication, is extremely important, especially treatments used even if the patient feels that they did not help. Be sure to ask about the use of antihistamines and about concordance with medications, and check inhaler and/or nasal spray technique if applicable.

Always check for a family history of atopy. Numerous research studies, including twin studies, have concluded that there is a clear genetic component in allergic diseases. With one atopic parent, a child has a 25–40% chance of being atopic themselves; this rises to a 70–80% chance if both parents are atopic.

Good history-taking must be coupled with a comprehensive examination.

2.2 Clinical examination in the allergic patient

Taking a detailed history may suggest areas of interest on which to focus the examination. Even if localising symptoms have not been reported in the history, it is good practice to check the skin, eyes, ear and throat in the allergic patient. It is important to check the entire respiratory system, nose and lungs.

Be on the lookout for the following signs and symptoms, which may indicate allergic conditions (see *Figure 2.2*):

- eyes – red, itchy eyes, epiphora and eyelid swelling
  note: these often co-exist with rhinitis, including in hayfever
- nose – watery rhinorrhoea, hyperaemic and congested nasal lining, nasal polyposis, hypertrophic turbinates
- chest – wheeze
- ear – a fluid level is seen behind the tympanic membrane, which may itself look grey/dull, visible air bubbles and, in severe cases, appear retracted
- skin – rash, red, blisters.

2.3 Investigations

Many investigations can be utilised to determine whether presenting symptoms are due to allergy. On the other hand, atopic individuals may have a positive skin-prick test or radioallergosorbent test (RAST) but may be asymptomatic. Therefore, without a suggestive history and the right test, clinical interpretation can be difficult.

Tests should be selected according to the merits of each case; tests that can be done in clinic, blood tests, laboratory tests and radiological imaging are all possibilities. Many can be carried out in-clinic before consultation with the specialist, for example peak nasal inspiratory flow, peak expiratory flow rate, spirometry and a skin-prick test for common airborne allergens, or can be arranged in advance of a clinic appointment, for example a RAST for specific allergens. Tests that can be carried out in-clinic are described individually below. These are useful in determining whether symptoms are due to atopy or not.

A battery of blood tests and provocation tests may be ordered after clinical consultation depending on its outcome – for further information see the sections below.

2.3.1 Nasal inspiratory peak flow

This test is done to assess the presence of obstruction in the nasal airway. It is performed using a peak nasal inspiratory flow meter (*Figure 2.3*), with calibration on one side of the device to record the readings.

It is important to educate the patient in the correct technique in order to obtain valid readings. These include ensuring nasal passages are as patent as possible (gently blowing the nose before they start) followed by removing glasses or anything else that may affect the seal of the device. Patients are advised to stand or sit up straight and, after exhaling, draw in a breath as sharply as they can. The breath is recorded in units of litres per minute (L/min) with the best of three readings recorded.

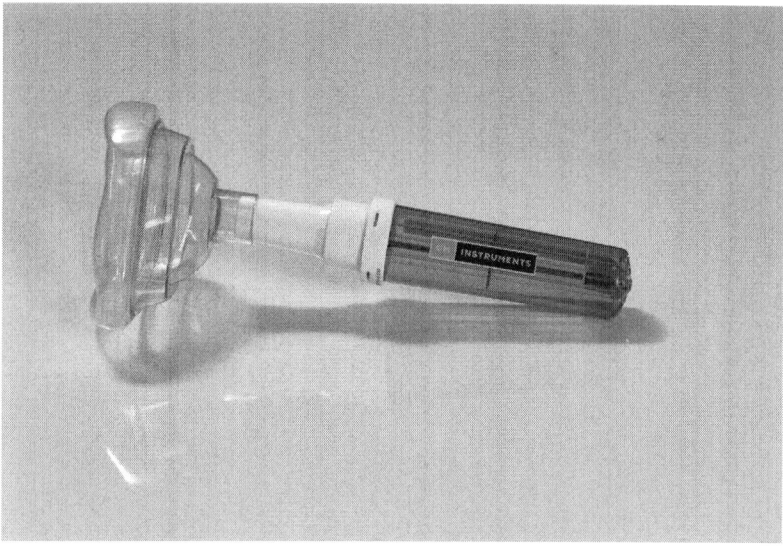

Figure 2.3 A peak nasal inspiratory flow meter. Photograph reproduced with permission from GM Instruments (www.gm-instruments.com).

2.3.2 Peak expiratory flow rate

This test has a similar purpose to that of peak nasal inspiratory flow; it is used to assess the airflow through the bronchial tree and thus the degree of obstruction in the airways.

Patients need to be educated as to the correct technique of use. The patient should be standing, holding the meter without obstructing the sliding scale in the middle, and should take a deep breath in, make a closed seal with their mouth around the end of the meter and then blow out into the meter as hard and as fast as they can. The best of three readings is recorded.

The peak expiratory flow rate is recorded in litres per minute (L/min) and assessed according to the patient's age, sex and height. Patients with obstructive airway disease can be asked to keep a regular peak flow diary, measuring twice a day to look for diurnal variation. The result of this test should considered in combination with the patient's symptoms.

2.3.3 Spirometry

Spirometry is important as an objective and complete measure of airflow limitation and of the possibility of reversibility in lung function after bronchodilator use (*Section 2.3.4, Pre- and post-bronchodilator spirometry*). The patient exhales into a spirometer; portable versions are available (*Figure 2.4*). The machine records values

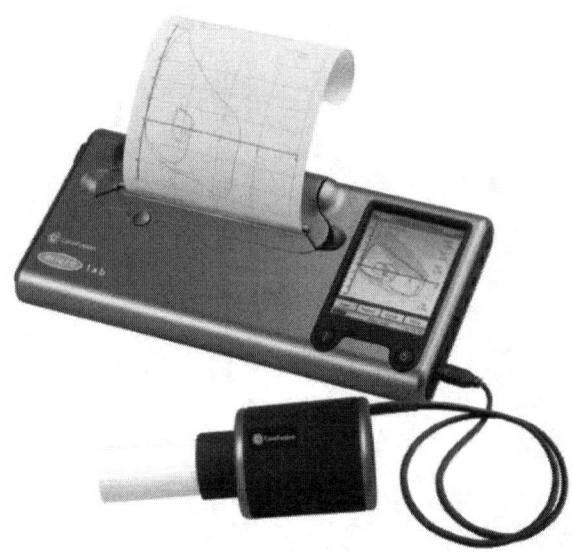

Figure 2.4 A portable spirometer. Image reproduced with permission from Becton, Dickinson UK Ltd.

on a graph of lung activity in the form of forced expiratory volume in 1 second (FEV_1) and forced vital capacity (FVC, the maximum volume of air that can be exhaled). This test can be used to confirm the diagnosis of asthma in individuals over the age of 5 years. The FEV_1/FVC ratio is normally greater than 70%; any value less than this suggests obstructive airway disease. In asthma, the result of spirometry can be normal when a patient is asymptomatic, whereas symptomatic asthma produces an obstructive picture.

2.3.4 Pre- and post-bronchodilator spirometry

This test can be performed on individuals aged 5 years or older by recording spirometry before and after administration of a bronchodilator.

If spirometry shows a FEV_1/FVC ratio less than 70%, then a bronchodilator in the form of a beta-2 agonist inhaler is given and after 20 minutes the lung function test is recorded again. An improvement of 12% or more in FEV_1 and an increase in lung capacity of 200 ml or more denote significant variability for which asthma should be considered as a cause. An improvement of greater than 400 ml in lung capacity is diagnostic of asthma.

2.3.5 Pre- and post-physical stimulus spirometry

For this test, spirometry is performed before and after patients perform vigorous physical exercise or are exposed to cold air, depending on what triggers their symptoms. This test can be performed if spirometry is normal but symptoms are suggestive of asthma.

Patients must discontinue long-acting medications 24 hours before the test according to medical advice. Tests of bronchial hyper-reactivity are contraindicated in patients with FEV_1 values less than 70% of the normal predicted value, patients with uncontrolled hypertension and patients who have recently experienced a stroke or a myocardial infarction.

2.3.6 Skin-prick test

The skin-prick test is the oldest form of allergy testing, first described in the mid-1800s. It is a minimally invasive and relatively inexpensive test. The results are available within a few minutes and, when carried out by trained healthcare professionals, are reproducible. Note that the healthcare professionals performing the test should be trained in resuscitation techniques.

Skin-prick testing can help to confirm the diagnosis of a suspected type I hypersensitivity. It can be used for a plethora of allergens – airborne allergens, pollens, foodstuffs, animal dander, mould and so on.

Some medications can interfere with the results of the test. Patients are advised to avoid antihistamines for the preceding 48–72 hours, as these alter the test result through changes in both IgE and IgG formation. Some tricyclic antidepressants can affect skin-prick test results and so it is recommended to stop these medications 2–4 days before a skin-prick test, but only after consultation with an appropriate healthcare professional.

The equipment required includes:
- allergen solutions or substances to be tested (should be within expiration date, as per instructions on the packaging)
- positive and negative control (histamine and diluent saline, respectively)
- lancets (one for each allergen and control)
- table to record results
- gauge to measure size of reaction
- sharps bin
- tissues.

Emergency equipment should be present and ready to use:
- antihistamine
- appropriate adrenaline auto-injector/solution
- inhalers: short-acting beta-2 agonist and inhaled corticosteroid
- hydrocortisone ointment
- calamine lotion.

The test involves pricking the skin with a small lancet at an angle of 90° (not deep enough to draw blood) on the volar surface of the patient's forearm to cause a localised allergic reaction. To begin, label areas of the volar surface with the allergen(s) to be tested. Ideally, sites should be spaced out by a minimum of 2 cm. If the positive reaction to the histamine control is placed too near other test sites it can initiate an axon reflex, which could drive the wheal-and-flare response. Apply a small drop of each allergen solution and of the positive and the negative control substance on the forearm, next to the respective label. If testing whole samples, such as fresh fruit or whole nuts, use the lancet to prick the substance and then the skin.

The patient should be advised that the area can become itchy and they should refrain from scratching.

The test results must be reviewed and interpreted 15–20 minutes after application. An example result is shown in *Figure 2.5*. A positive result (confirming sensitisation) is defined as a wheal (the raised area in the centre of the test site, with the erythema around the raised area defined as a flare) with a mean diameter more than 3 mm wider than the negative control. The mean diameter is recorded by measuring the largest diameter and the diameters at right angles to it, adding them and dividing by 2. The measurement excludes pseudopodia (the tails of the reaction, although note their presence). The results of skin-prick testing should be interpreted in the context of patient's history.

False positives and negatives can occur. A negative reaction to the positive control may signify antihistamine intake in the preceding 48–72 hours. The negative control helps provide evidence for sensitisation and helps exclude the presence of dermographism, in which skin is over-responsive to minor trauma, causing a wheal response to the negative control. Patients who become symptomatic during the pollen season can be more sensitive to skin-prick tests done during this time.

The preferred documentation method is to copy the outline of the wheal onto translucent cellophane tape and stick the tape onto the skin-prick test result sheet.

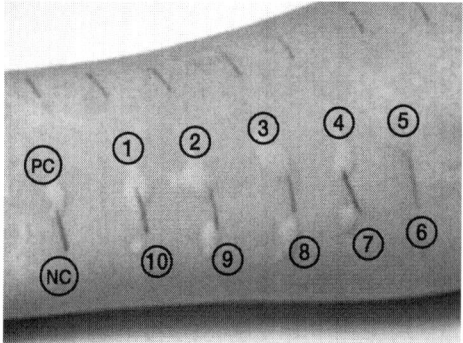

Figure 2.5 A typical skin-prick test to a range of animals (1–5), *Alternaria* fungal mould (6), and a range of pollens (7–10); a positive control (PC) and negative control (NC) are also included. Positive results were seen to all pollens and all animals except for sheep wool (at 5); there was also a negative result to *Alternaria* mould (at 6).

2.3.7 Blood tests

These tests should be requested given an appropriate history. They involve a trained phlebotomist taking a sample of blood from the individual.

Haematology and biochemistry

Tests include:
- full blood count
- erythrocyte sedimentation rate
- C-reactive protein
- urea and electrolytes
- thyroid function test including autoantibodies
- liver function tests.

Specialist tests include:
- angiotensin-converting enzyme (ACE) level
- antineutrophil cytoplasmic antibodies
- total IgG
- IgE level
- *Aspergillus* precipitin.

Eosinophilia (an absolute eosinophil count of 5×10^8/L or higher) is associated with allergic conditions. Not all of the tests above are aimed at identifying atopic disease, but they are important nonetheless to allow for identification or exclusion of other causes.

Serum mast-cell tryptase

This test is helpful after an anaphylactic reaction, as it can remain transiently raised for up to 6 hours after the event. However, a normal result at the time does not rule anaphylaxis out.

Immunoglobulin assay

This automated test assesses the levels of antibody present within the blood.

Allergen-specific IgE

This test measures the levels of IgE antibodies to specific allergens; it can provide an indication as to what is triggering the body's reaction.

Radioallergosorbent test (RAST) and enzyme-linked immunosorbent assay (ELISA) testing

In the RAST, the suspected allergen, fixed to an insoluble substrate, is treated with serum from the patient followed by radioactively labelled anti-human antibodies. If radioactivity is detected after rinsing the substrate, the specific IgE must have been present in the plasma to bind to the allergen.

As radioactivity poses a potential health threat, a safer alternative was sought. In an ELISA test, an enzyme-activated marker is used to bind to captured antibodies. If any bound enzyme is present, the final stage of the test causes a detectable change in the test solution, analysis of which involves measuring the amount of IgG.

RAST and ELISA tests can be used to test for inhalant allergies, insect sting allergies and some food sensitivities. They cannot be used to reveal the severity of reactions that a patient has experienced or is likely to experience in the future.

2.3.8 Laboratory and challenge tests

These tests are done by specialists with experience in this field. Where appropriate, emergency treatment should be available, with suitably trained healthcare professionals present.

Fraction exhaled nitric oxide (FeNO)

The FeNO test is available in specialist clinics or laboratories. Individuals with allergic inflammation of the airways exhale a higher level of nitric oxide in their breath than unaffected individuals. Evidence suggests that exhaled nitric oxide levels can be used to support the diagnosis of asthma, determine whether patients will respond to steroid therapy and monitor patient response to asthma therapy.

The patient exhales into a handheld device. To correctly carry out the test the patient must first exhale into the air (to eliminate any environmental NO), make a tight seal with their mouth over the mouthpiece of the machine, take a deep breath in and then exhale into the machine. In children aged under 5 an alternative, shorter version of the test can be performed. The machine records the concentration of exhaled nitric oxide.

A result of a level above 40 parts per billion (ppb) is considered a positive in adult patients who are not using inhaled corticosteroids. In children aged 5 years onwards, a result of 35 ppb is considered a positive result. Results should only be interpreted in the context of the history, examination and other test findings.

Nasal eosinophil smear

This test can substantiate the diagnosis of allergic rhinitis. The smear can be taken during nasal examination, with the patient's consent, and sent to a laboratory to determine eosinophil levels. Raised eosinophil levels can indicate local allergic rhinitis.

Patch test

In clinical practice, a patient suspected of having allergic contact dermatitis or atopic dermatitis should receive patch testing. This is because these allergens may cause a delayed allergic reaction, which follows the type IV hypersensitivity pattern and may not be identified by blood testing or skin-prick testing.

The patch test produces local allergic reactions on a test area on a patient's back. The allergens are prepared in a patch-test kit as tiny quantities in individual chambers that are applied to the patient's back and kept in place with hypoallergenic tape labelled with a marker pen. Approximately 40 allergens are commonly used in patch testing, although the allergens are selected on a case-by-case basis.

Patch tests are conducted over three hospital visits. The first visit involves application of the allergens to the patient's back. On the second visit the next day the tape is removed and the skin inspected to see whether any reactions are present. During the third visit, the day after the second, the patient's back will be examined and results noted and discussed. Results can be expressed as negative, equivocal or uncertain, weak positive, strong positive and extreme reactions.

In some cases, if a reaction related to exposure to sunlight is suspected, the skin is also exposed to long-wavelength ultraviolet light. This is called photo-patch testing.

Specific challenge tests

Challenge tests are used to confirm allergy and reactions to specific substances. Commonly tested substances include:
- aspirin
- foodstuffs
- animal allergens.

These tests must be performed in a hospital environment where emergency equipment and trained staff are available. They should not be attempted in patients with a history of anaphylaxis.

The **aspirin challenge** is performed by introducing aspirin in a controlled environment and recording potential reactions. It is strongly recommended that this test should be done in hospital, by specialists where emergency equipment is available.

Food challenges require that the patient abstains from the food suspected of causing allergy for 72 hours (though this depends on the institution delivering the test) and from antihistamine for a similar period. The suspect foodstuff is then reintroduced in the controlled setting of the hospital, where reactions can be recorded and there are sufficient resources to respond to emergencies. This test should be avoided, or considered as a last resort, in suspected severe food allergies.

A **nasal provocation challenge** gives a true reflection of the response of the nasal mucosa to specific allergens. Again, it should be performed in hospital under the supervision of an allergy specialist.

The **methacholine challenge or bronchial provocation test** is carried out in a hospital respiratory lab where emergency medicines and care are available. It is not a routine test. Methacholine is a known asthma trigger: when inhaled it can cause contraction of the airway. This test is performed if, despite other tests, the diagnosis remains uncertain. Spirometry is performed before and after inhalation of methacholine. A 20% drop in FEV_1 is regarded as significant. Caffeine-containing substances, smoking and exercise should be avoided before the test; institutions have their own guidelines regarding timing, but the range is from hours to a day beforehand.

2.4 Radiological imaging

In the case of nasal and sinus symptoms, especially those not responding to treatment, a computed tomography (CT) scan of the nose and sinuses should be considered.

The optimal imaging modalities to investigate lung pathology are either a chest radiograph or, if indicated, a chest CT scan.

Chapter 3
Clinical allergy

3.1	Systemic allergy	34
3.2	Skin allergies	39
3.3	Eye	41
3.4	Nose and sinus	42
3.5	Ear	44
3.6	Respiratory	44
3.7	Food and oral allergies	46
3.8	Drug allergy	50
3.9	Latex allergy	51
3.10	Insect allergy	51
3.11	Others	52

3.1 Systemic allergy

3.1.1 Anaphylaxis

Anaphylaxis is a severe, life-threatening, systemic allergic reaction affecting multiple organ systems. It is an example of a type I hypersensitivity reaction and is a **medical emergency**. After exposure to an allergen, IgE specific to the allergen encountered causes huge degranulation of mast cells (this mechanism is described in *Section 1.5, What is hypersensitivity?*).

Symptoms are acute, and may include:
- bronchospasm –shortness of breath, wheeze, cyanosis
- systemic hypotension – collapse, tachycardia
- angioedema of the face and tongue (can also affect the larynx, resulting in stridor)
- cutaneous manifestations – urticaria, pruritus, erythema
- gastrointestinal manifestations – nausea, vomiting, diarrhoea, abdominal pain.

Causes

Common anaphylaxis-causing substances may be foods, including peanuts (a legume), tree nuts, fish, shellfish, sesame, eggs and dairy products, and non-food substances, such as insect stings (wasp and bee), medications (including some antibiotics and contrast dye used in radiological imaging) and latex.

In some cases, an anaphylactic reaction may occur when allergen exposure occurs alongside a second provoker, e.g. exercise or certain drugs such as aspirin.

Diagnosis

The history is key to determining the chronological course of events, which can help to confirm the diagnosis of anaphylaxis and eliminate other plausible diagnoses, as well as suggesting the probable trigger. It is important to stress here that an individual has to have been sensitised through prior exposure, described in *Section 1.5, What is hypersensitivity?*. Do not be afraid to go into detail about all recent exposures, if necessary.

Blood tests for mast-cell tryptase can be useful in confirming the type of reaction occurring (though a normal reading does not exclude anaphylaxis). Mast-cell tryptase level remains elevated for 6 hours (some sources say for longer). Current NICE guideline on anaphylaxis (2011, CG134) advises taking two samples, one as soon as the acute event commences and another 1–2 hours later but no more than 4 hours after the event has started.

Anaphylactic reactions are typically graded as mild, moderate or severe (but note

that any anaphylaxis reaction is potentially life-threatening).
- Mild reactions can involve urticaria, pruritus, erythema, mild angioedema, conjunctivitis and rhinitis.
- Moderate reactions can include mild asthma, moderate angioedema, abdominal pain, vomiting, diarrhoea and minor hypotensive symptoms such as light-headedness and dizziness.
- Severe reactions can involve respiratory difficulty e.g. asthma or laryngeal oedema, hypotension, collapse or loss of consciousness, faecal and urinary incontinence, seizures.

There is a risk that symptoms will recur after recovery from the initial event despite no further exposure to the allergen. Such a recurrence usually happens within 72 hours, and unfortunately there is no way of predicting whether a patient will experience it; see *Section 1.5.1, Type I reaction*.

Skin-prick testing and challenge testing can be performed in extreme cases, keeping in mind that they can cause further systemic reactions. They should be used with extreme caution and only with experts at hand and cardiopulmonary resuscitation equipment immediately available.

Management

An ABCDE (airway, breathing, circulation, disability and exposure) approach is used in the recognition and treatment of anaphylactic reaction. Immediate management involves administering adrenaline, given as an intramuscular (IM) injection unless you are experienced with intravenous (IV) administration. IM adrenaline is given, repeated after every 5 minutes if symptoms do not improve. The dosages of adrenaline are indicated in the Resuscitation Council (UK) guidelines shown in *Figure 3.1* (always check for updated guidelines).

If the skills and equipment are available, further actions to take unless contraindicated (*Figure 3.1*) are administration of:
- IV fluid challenge (maintain blood pressure)
- chlorphenamine (antihistamine)
- hydrocortisone (steroid, for treating a potential late-phase reaction).

Again, check Resuscitation Council (UK) guidelines for the most recent treatment algorithm.

If an individual is at risk of having an anaphylactic reaction, they should be given an adrenaline auto-injector to be kept for their own use (commonly called an EpiPen©) and counselling on how to use it. Currently, 0.3 mg and 0.15 mg strength auto-injectors are available (although there is worldwide shortage at the time of writing (December 2019)).

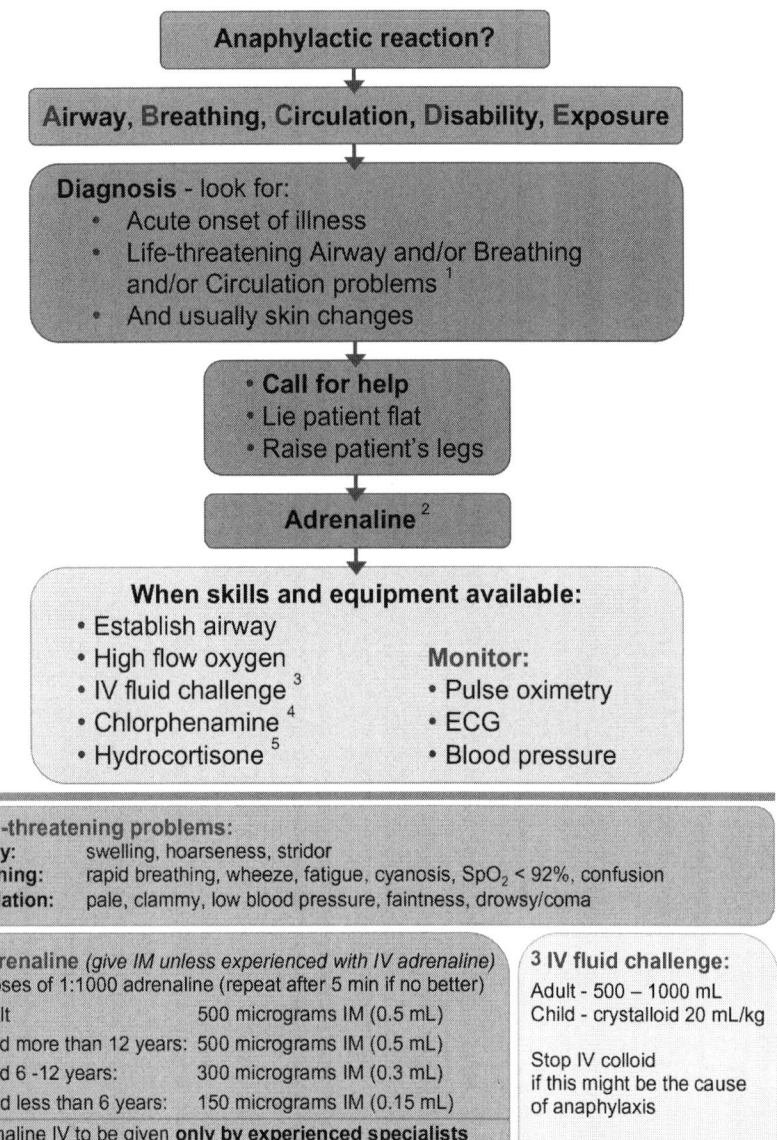

Anaphylactic reaction?

Airway, Breathing, Circulation, Disability, Exposure

Diagnosis - look for:
- Acute onset of illness
- Life-threatening Airway and/or Breathing and/or Circulation problems [1]
- And usually skin changes

- **Call for help**
- Lie patient flat
- Raise patient's legs

Adrenaline [2]

When skills and equipment available:
- Establish airway
- High flow oxygen
- IV fluid challenge [3]   **Monitor:**
- Chlorphenamine [4]   - Pulse oximetry
- Hydrocortisone [5]   - ECG
                              - Blood pressure

[1] **Life-threatening problems:**
Airway: swelling, hoarseness, stridor
Breathing: rapid breathing, wheeze, fatigue, cyanosis, SpO_2 < 92%, confusion
Circulation: pale, clammy, low blood pressure, faintness, drowsy/coma

[2] **Adrenaline** *(give IM unless experienced with IV adrenaline)*
IM doses of 1:1000 adrenaline (repeat after 5 min if no better)
- Adult   500 micrograms IM (0.5 mL)
- Child more than 12 years: 500 micrograms IM (0.5 mL)
- Child 6 -12 years: 300 micrograms IM (0.3 mL)
- Child less than 6 years: 150 micrograms IM (0.15 mL)

Adrenaline IV to be given **only by experienced specialists**
Titrate: Adults 50 micrograms; Children 1 microgram/kg

[3] **IV fluid challenge:**
Adult - 500 – 1000 mL
Child - crystalloid 20 mL/kg

Stop IV colloid
if this might be the cause
of anaphylaxis

	[4] Chlorphenamine (IM or slow IV)	[5] Hydrocortisone (IM or slow IV)
Adult or child more than 12 years	10 mg	200 mg
Child 6 - 12 years	5 mg	100 mg
Child 6 months to 6 years	2.5 mg	50 mg
Child less than 6 months	250 micrograms/kg	25 mg

Figure 3.1 Anaphylaxis protocol. Reproduced with permission from the Resuscitation Council (UK).

Patients should be observed for 6 to 12 hours from symptom onset. Those under 16 years of age should be admitted under the paediatric medical team. If the reaction was easily controlled and treatment has been effective, however, the assessing physician may decide on a shorter observation period.

It is important to provide patients with information about their condition, including support groups (organisations recognised by NICE are the Anaphylaxis Campaign, Allergy UK and the Latex Allergy Support Group), the allergen(s) they must avoid and what to do if they do come into contact with the allergen, and the possibility of a biphasic reaction. This is known as an 'allergy action plan'. It is important to tell patients to call the emergency services even if self-administered adrenaline provides relief.

Patients who have had an anaphylactic reaction should be followed up in allergy clinic.

3.1.2 Anaphylactoid reactions

These reactions are clinically similar to anaphylaxis; however, mast-cell degranulation is IgE-independent. It occurs either through direct activation of mast cells or through indirect pathways.

Causes

Substances causing anaphylactoid reactions include:
- drugs: opioids, cyclo-oxygenase inhibitors, non-steroidal anti-inflammatory drugs (NSAIDs), vancomycin, thiamine, some contrast agents (preventative measures can be taken to avoid these reactions, see *Management* below), some anaesthetics, intravenous immunoglobulins and some blood products
- foods: strawberries, ingestion of oily fish that has been decomposed by bacteria (ultimately leads to excess histamine release)
- physical stimuli: trauma, exercise, low temperatures.

Diagnosis

The history is important, and tryptase levels will be elevated. No allergen-specific IgE will be detectable.

Management

Acute management is as for that of anaphylaxis, see *Section 3.1.1* above.

In those known to react to intravenous contrast medium, low osmolality dyes should be considered to prevent reaction (lower incidence) and oral corticosteroids, with an antihistamine and a histamine receptor blocker, can be given before the procedure (check local guidelines for precise medications and dosage).

3.1.3 Angioedema

Angioedema is a swelling of deep tissue, causing pressure discomfort, which can affect any part of the body. The production of bradykinin, through activation of the kinin system, is thought to be the mechanism behind this response. Sometimes, a tingling sensation can be felt before the swelling occurs.

Causes

Angioedema may be hereditary or acquired. Hereditary angioedema is inherited in an autosomal-dominant fashion and usually affects older children/teenagers in flares. It is caused by a deficiency or reduced function of C1 esterase inhibitor. It is not associated with urticaria.

Angioedema can also be a standalone response to a stimulus (not IgE-mediated). It can be due to medication, including ACE inhibitors (less so with angiotensin II receptor blockers), NSAIDs, aspirin (the latter two are known to cause urticarial angioedema) and statins.

It can also be part of the allergic response; see *Section 3.1.1*.

Diagnosis

It is important to recognise whether the angioedema is part of an allergic response. The history is key in determining this.

Hereditary angioedema comes in 'attacks' usually manifesting as cutaneous (especially peripheral), intestinal or laryngeal oedema, the last being the least common but most severe. It is often fleeting and affects different sites in each attack.

Management

When part of the allergic response, angioedema can be accompanied by other features including anaphylaxis and urticaria. Severe swelling of the tongue is considered a medical emergency because of the risk to the airway.

If anaphylaxis is present, then it should be treated as described earlier (see *Section 3.1.1*).

Specific management of angioedema involves trigger avoidance and long-acting antihistamines as prophylaxis.

Hereditary angioedema has its own treatment pathway and should be managed by specialists. Prophylactic treatment with danazol (or tranexamic acid) is available. Other options, especially in acute attacks, include C1 esterase inhibitor, fresh frozen plasma or a bradykinin beta-2 receptor antagonist.

3.2 Skin allergies

3.2.1 Atopic eczema

This is one of the most common presentations of allergy, and is increasing in prevalence. It typically presents in childhood. It tends to affect the face and trunk in children and the flexor regions in older sufferers. It can be associated with other forms of allergic diseases such as allergic asthma, allergic rhinitis and contact dermatitis (for which it is a risk factor).

Note that children diagnosed in the first year of life usually grow out of the condition by the age of 14 years.

Causes

The role of the type I hypersensitivity reaction in atopic eczema is still unclear, with evidence for the type IV reaction contributing as type 2 T helper cells (see *Section 1.4.4, Lymphocytes*) infiltrate the skin.

In atopic eczema, susceptibility to itch is increased, which can result in lichenification of the eczematous areas of skin. During this chronic phase, inflammatory cells including mast cells, eosinophils and basophils are all upregulated in the skin.

Diagnosis

As is the case with allergic disease, the history is key in determining the cause. Atopic eczema is present if there is a history of itchy skin along with at least three of the following:
- history of asthma or allergic rhinitis
- history of dry skin within the last year
- either visible or history of dermatitis in flexor regions
- onset of symptoms under the age of 2.

Concomitant infections (e.g. warts, molluscum contagiosum and eczema herpeticum) alongside the above-mentioned symptoms are commonly present alongside atopic eczema.

On blood testing, eosinophilia with high levels of IgE is a common finding. Skin-prick testing can identify specific IgE.

Management

The management of atopic eczema differs for those over the age of 12 and those younger. Management in children under 12 is discussed in *Chapter 8, Allergy in children*.

It is important to gauge the impact of the symptoms on the patient's quality of life in order to maintain a patient-centred approach to care. Though in most cases the disease is mild, some patients may experience significant consequences for their psychological wellbeing and confidence; adequate support should be provided in these domains.

For patients over the age of 12, first-line treatment consists of emollients (use liberally), soap substitutes and topical corticosteroid therapy. Antihistamines can help reduce itching. Also note that some non-specific irritants (such as stress, heat or wool) can exacerbate the problem.

Options for further treatment depend upon the age of the patient. For those aged 12–16, topical tacrolimus (within its clinical indications) is an option for moderate to severe atopic eczema. Pimecrolimus is also an option, to be used on the face and neck. In adults with moderate to severe atopic eczema, dupilumab can be considered if the disease has not responded to at least one other systemic therapy, or other therapies are not tolerated/are contraindicated. Dupilumab should be stopped at 16 weeks if there has not been an adequate response (local guidelines should be checked for the definition of an adequate response). Topical tacrolimus (within its clinical indications) is an option in adults too.

For adults with chronic severe hand eczema, alitretinoin can be used if the patient has not responded to potent topical corticosteroids. This treatment should be stopped once an adequate response has been achieved, or if an adequate response has not been achieved by 24 weeks or the eczema remains severe at 12 weeks.

3.2.2 Contact dermatitis (hypersensitivity)

This is a localised type IV hypersensitivity reaction (see *Section 1.5*), which is due to contact with an allergen. It typically presents as an eczematous rash with blistering. Sensitisation occurs before reactivity.

Causes

Sources of allergic contact dermatitis include:
- metals, e.g. nickel, cobalt, chromium
- rubber – latex and synthetic forms
- cosmetics, e.g. fragrances and hair dyes
- aniline dyes – in leather and cloth
- resins
- drugs, e.g. gentamicin.

Some allergens also require sun exposure to react, and so will only present in sun-exposed locations of the body. Examples of such allergens include plants (such as meadow-grass) and some drugs (such as tetracyclines and sulfonamides).

Diagnosis

The history and examination are key to diagnosis. It is important to note that irritants such as acid and alkali can cause a similar presentation termed 'irritant dermatitis', and history-taking should permit differentiation of the two.

Patch testing can be used to aid diagnosis.

Management

Antihistamines can be used as a control measure for the sensation of itch. Potent topical steroids should provide relief in combination with allergen avoidance. In cases of nickel sensitivity, treatment should be supplemented with a low-nickel diet. Foodstuffs high in nickel are commonly available, e.g. chocolate, certain wheat bran, canned food as well as vitamins supplemented with nickel.

3.3 Eye

3.3.1 Allergic conjunctivitis

Allergic conjunctivitis often co-exists with rhinitis, thanks to the nasolacrimal duct and similar mechanisms. It can have a significant impact, especially on students studying or sitting examinations in the summer, hence needs to be promptly identified and appropriately addressed.

Causes

Common triggers include pollen, animal dander and dust mites.

Diagnosis

History is significant, especially in the context of the symptoms of a watery, itching eye with redness and possibly swelling of the eyelids.

Eosinophilia is not always present; however, a skin-prick test (correlated with indications from the history) will be helpful.

Management

Treatment options include topical antihistamines and mast-cell stabilising agents (including sodium cromoglicate, nedocromil and lodoxamide, which is specifically for allergic eye conditions). Severe symptoms can be treated with oral antihistamines.

Topical steroids may be prescribed by ophthalmologists, who will monitor the patient because of the risk of glaucoma and cataracts when steroids are used in the long term. If topical therapies do not provide adequate relief, the next step can include a short course of oral steroids.

3.4 Nose and sinus

3.4.1 Allergic rhinitis

Rhinitis can have allergic or non-allergic aetiology. The allergic variants typically present as either seasonal or perennial, with patients describing symptoms of rhinorrhoea, itching, sneezing and/or nasal congestion.

Rhinitis strictly means inflammation of the nasal lining, but seldom occurs without some degree of involvement of the sinus lining, termed rhinosinusitis. Associated symptoms in the eyes (see *Section 3.3.1*) and throat can also occur.

Causes

Typical causative agents, which can be identified with skin-prick testing, include:
- grass pollens (typically presents late spring to early summer)
- tree pollens (typically presents in spring)
- house dust mite (symptoms worse on waking and in the winter, but can present year-round)
- animal dander (all year round with exposure to animal)
- weed pollens (typically presents from early spring to late autumn)
- occupational (symptoms may be alleviated during time off work, e.g. weekends or holidays)
- moulds (all year round, but worse in winter).

Diagnosis

The history, alongside examination of the nasal cavity, is important. Timing of symptoms and temporal association with exposure to an allergen are indicative. Patients with allergic rhinitis usually present at around 7 years of age, and it persists into adulthood. Consider the diagnosis if other causes of rhinitis have been excluded.

It is important to remember that patients may seek first-line over-the-counter help, not necessarily presenting to primary care immediately at symptom onset, so be sure to ask about previous treatments. Often patients present to primary care only when symptoms stop responding or quality of life is affected, so it is important to assess the impact of their symptoms in this regard.

Check for sinus (rhinosinusitis) and eye symptoms. Be sure to ask about other atopic disease and family history of atopy.

Skin-prick testing can be used to determine sensitivity to specific allergens (see *Causes*, above).

A test for specific IgE in the serum can be carried out in young children or in those in whom skin-prick testing is contraindicated.

Management

Allergen avoidance techniques can be suggested where possible. For example, in grass pollen allergy, patients should avoid walking in grassy areas and keep house and car windows shut when there is a high pollen count.

In house dust mite allergy, patients should use cotton bedding and wet mopping, avoid keeping furry toys, ideally have no carpets and have blinds instead of curtains fitted to windows.

In animal allergy, ideally exposure should be limited by not keeping animals at home; if this is not possible then restrict animal contact in the house by keeping them in one or two rooms only and washing the animals and cleaning those areas regularly.

In occupational allergy, relocation may not always be possible, so patients should be advised to ensure adequate ventilation in their working space and to use respiratory protection such as facemasks. If items of use in the workplace are the source of the allergy, then alternatives should be offered and exposure minimised.

In terms of pharmacological treatment, patients should be advised to take medication at periods of exposure to allergens; in the case of perennial allergic rhinitis this may mean ongoing treatment. If symptoms persist a fortnight to a month after treatment is initiated, then a review is needed.

It is vital that correct technique for using nasal therapies is practised to maximise the chances of the treatment working effectively.

Pharmacological treatment (*Table 3.1*) for mild to moderate intermittent or mild persistent symptoms includes either intranasal (first-line) or oral antihistamines as and when required. If these are contraindicated, intranasal chromones can be considered.

Table 3.1 Optimal medication depending on predominant symptom. +, relative effectiveness in improving the symptom; –, little or no benefit; LTRA, leukotriene receptor antagonist.

Symptom \ Medication	Antihistamine	Cromoglicate	LTRA	Anticholinergic	Decongestant	Steroid
Itching	+++	+++	+	–	–	++
Sneezing	+++	+/–	+	–	–	++
Rhinorrhoea	+/–	+/–	+	+++	+/–	+++
Blocked nose	–	–	+/–	–	+++	+++
Swollen lining	–	–	–	–	–	+++

Nasal irrigation with saline can be suggested to patients as an option that may offer some symptom relief.

In moderate to severe persistent symptoms, or if initial therapy has failed, then regular intranasal corticosteroids can be used in periods of allergen exposure. Nasal steroids are especially helpful if nasal obstruction is a major symptom; in this case, they can be used earlier.

Immunotherapy may be suitable for some patients with allergic rhinitis, but should be considered only by specialists with experience.

Because effective symptomatic treatment (especially steroid-based nasal therapies or antihistamines) are available in primary care, many patients may not return for a review or further investigations. This takes away the opportunity to devise a definitive management plan by weighing up the long-term risks and benefits of such therapies as well as the use of novel therapies. On the other hand, some patients concordant on treatment and allergen avoidance remain symptomatic.

If complications such as allergic nasal polyposis are present, a specialist opinion will be required.

3.5 Ear

3.5.1 Secretory otitis media ('glue ear')

'Glue ear' can develop as a complication of atopic disease such as allergic rhinitis. The condition was proved to be a complication of allergic disease when histamine was found in the middle ear fluid. In such cases the allergy may present as recurrent ear infections, potentially affecting the child's hearing and speech. The history may alert you to ear pathology (for example, presence of nasal obstruction, rhinorrhoea, sleep apnoea, or recurrent ear infections), and examination should identify relevant physical signs.

If suspected, necessary investigations should be requested and management subsequently commenced accordingly (see *ENT Made Easy* for further details). In short, patients will need a hearing test such as an audiogram, middle-ear pressure test such as a tympanogram, and a skin-prick test/RAST.

3.6 Respiratory

For asthma, see *Chapter 4*.

3.6.1 Hypersensitivity pneumonitis

Hypersensitivity pneumonitis, formerly termed extrinsic allergic alveolitis, is based on a delayed reaction to the repetitive inhalation of allergens by sensitised individuals; the delay is by approximately 6 hours. The response is a type III hypersensitivity reaction; there may be some degree of type IV involvement as well.

There are acute (inflammatory cell infiltrate in the alveoli) and chronic (granuloma formation and obliterative bronchiolitis) forms of the condition.

A variety of occupations can be affected, including farmers, brewers and bird breeders.

Causes

The most common causes in the UK are:
- avian proteins (commonly pigeons)
- thermophilic fungi on farms.

In many chronic cases, no cause can be identified.

Diagnosis

A history of allergen exposure coupled with a typical presentation should help to identify the condition.

In the acute state, patients complain of dyspnoea, a dry cough and flu-like symptoms, usually within 4–6 hours of exposure. Auscultation reveals fine crackles on the chest bibasally.

In the chronic state, patients complain of worsening dyspnoea and weight loss. Examination may reveal clubbing (in approximately half of all patients) with acute hypoxaemia. Some may develop cor pulmonale. This usually occurs after years of exposure.

Acutely, blood tests may reveal a raised *Aspergillus* precipitin and raised IgG. Chest radiography may show pulmonary infiltrate. The use of bronchoalveolar lavage can differentiate this condition from other similar presentations, on the basis of lymphocytosis and increased cytotoxic T cells.

Management

Although steroids can be used for the management of symptoms (both acute and chronic), avoidance of the allergen is critical for optimal disease management. Irreversible damage can occur with continued exposure, and this should be made clear to the patient. Acutely, provided there is no further exposure, resolution can occur within a couple of days; hence it is important to develop a shared management plan with the patient on how to avoid exposure.

If the patient is hypoxic, supplemental oxygen can be provided.

In the UK, compensation may be sought for chronic cases according to the National Insurance (Industrial Injuries) Act 1965.

3.6.2 Allergic bronchopulmonary aspergillosis

Allergic bronchopulmonary aspergillosis is a specific entity that results from allergy to the fungus *Aspergillus*. It is both a type I and a type III hypersensitivity reaction. It is more common in the context of an underlying (yet advanced) lung disorder, such as cystic fibrosis or asthma (more so in the former) when there is a history of atopy.

Blood tests will again show a raised precipitin but this time there will also be a raised total IgE and, in an acute episode, there is a marked eosinophilia. Sputum will usually be culture-positive for *Aspergillus*. Skin-prick testing will be strongly positive to *Aspergillus*.

Treatment involves corticosteroid therapy for acute treatment; some cases need continuous low-dose therapy once symptoms resolve. Bronchodilators may be required, as bronchiectasis can develop.

3.7 Food and oral allergies

3.7.1 Food allergy

Food allergy is an adverse immunologic response to a food protein. It is estimated that 6–8% of children under the age of 5 years experience food allergies and (as some children 'grow out' of their allergies) approximately 3–4% of adults. Food allergies evoke reactions of varying severity, from cutaneous responses only through to life-threatening anaphylactic reactions.

Abnormal reactions to food ingestion have many possible causes, listed below. It is important to carefully assess the patient for food poisoning.

- Food poisoning: a reaction caused by endotoxins or exotoxins in the food or released by contaminating micro-organisms; an example of the latter occurs when bacteria in spoiled food convert the amino acid histidine, found in the food (particularly fish), into histamine; the histamine, when consumed in large quantities, causes a reaction in the individual
- Enzyme deficiency: for example, lactose intolerance is caused by lactase deficiency, broad beans trigger haemolysis in people with glucose-6-phosphate dehydrogenase deficiency, and aldehyde dehydrogenase deficiency results in flushing and discomfort on consumption of alcohol
- Intrinsic gastrointestinal pathology such as coeliac disease (autoimmune condition)
- Reaction to food additives ('E-numbers') in food and drinks, which can cause allergy-like symptoms
- Direct effects of the foodstuffs: for example, caffeine is a stimulant, therefore can cause symptoms of shaking and tachycardia; tyramine in aged cheese can cause headaches.

Food allergy can occur by all four immunological hypersensitivity mechanisms (see *Section 1.5, What is hypersensitivity?*). We will discuss it in terms of IgE-mediated and non-IgE-mediated reactions.

IgE-mediated allergies appear within seconds to a few minutes of exposure to the allergen, are referred to as 'fixed food allergy' and represent 5–20% of all food hypersensitivity. There is a greater risk of anaphylaxis with this type of allergy. The late-phase type I reaction can be seen in asthma, and its mechanism is still a subject of research.

In non-IgE-mediated food allergies, symptoms take longer to develop and the allergies are more difficult to diagnose. Many non-IgE reactions, which are poorly defined both clinically and scientifically, are believed to be T-cell-mediated. Some reactions involve a mixture of both IgE and non-IgE responses and are classified as mixed IgE and non-IgE allergic reactions. They usually present as symptoms of the gastrointestinal system, skin and/or respiratory system.

Fixed food allergy is rapid onset and severe in intensity. Cyclic reactions (see *Section 1.5.5, Fixed and cyclic types*) can be immediate or delayed (from hours to 3–4 days). These reactions can be dose- and frequency-related: the more frequently food is ingested, the more pronounced and rapid the response will be.

Causes

In food allergy, an allergenic protein in food survives food preparation, stomach acid and bodily enzymes to ultimately be absorbed from the gastrointestinal tract and subsequently cause an allergic reaction. Theoretically, all foodstuffs can be the source of allergy. Food allergies can be caused by foods in one state and not in another; that is, a food may be allergenic in its raw state but not when cooked or vice versa. In particular this can be the case in fruit and vegetable allergies.

Table 3.2 is a list of food allergies by age. Common allergies include: eggs, milk, nuts (including peanuts, although technically these are legumes), seafood (including shellfish), soybeans, wheat, some fruits (including citrus and berries), celery and melon.

Table 3.2 Examples of common food allergies, split by prevalence in children and adults

Adults	Children
Nuts: peanuts, tree nuts	Milk
	Eggs
Fruits	Peanuts
Fish	Tree nuts
Shellfish	Fish
Soya	Shellfish
Wheat	Soya

Diagnosis

The history is vital, even though the symptoms of food allergy can be vague and can affect many systems – for example, from vague itching in the mouth/throat/eye to vomiting, diarrhoea and abdominal cramps. It can even cause earaches, eczema and migraine. It can induce anaphylaxis (see *Section 3.1.1*). This all needs to be put into context of a detailed history, also including a history of other allergic diseases such as eczema, skin rash, asthma, rhinitis and/or conjunctivitis, followed by a clinical examination.

Investigations should be chosen according to the history and results of the examination. Skin-prick testing is a safe, sensitive and rapid method for IgE-mediated food allergy. This test has 90% sensitivity, while specificity is 50%. If skin-prick testing cannot be done, then a RAST (see *Section 2.3*) can be done to diagnose food allergy. Where necessary and safe to do so, a food challenge (in the hospital setting) can be carried out (see *Section 2.3*).

Management

Management begins with ensuring the allergy is a true food allergy; a food symptom diary with special attention to the suspected food allergen may be kept. A food elimination diet can be used for both diagnosis and treatment of food allergy – initially eliminate the food for 2 weeks, with subsequent reintroduction of the eliminated food. The patient should continue to keep a food symptom diary. Dietitian advice and review by an allergist are important.

Once a true food allergy has been identified, management involves patient education, as the mainstay of treatment is avoidance. Again, specialist dietary support should be sought. Antihistamines are usually not needed regularly, but can be advised as a prophylactic measure.

Patients who have experienced anaphylaxis and those at risk of anaphylactic reactions need to be given adrenaline auto-injectors alongside an action plan about usage, training on how to use the auto-injectors and education about their allergy.

Immunotherapy is also possible in some cases, hence the input of an allergy specialist is important. There are a variety of different methods, and varied licences and commissioning methods apply for the medications. Given the fast-paced progress of this therapy, it is best to review the latest recommendations at the time of the patient's assessment.

3.7.2 Contact allergy to food

Some foods can cause a contact-allergy type picture, in which exposure is not limited to ingestion only: for example, those sensitised to peanuts may develop an erythematous rash or angioedema from even minimal contact. The history and presentation of the rash will point towards this cause. Patch testing or further specialist testing may be required.

3.7.3 Oral allergy syndrome

Oral allergy syndrome (OAS) is a comparatively newly recognised condition in which patients with tree or grass pollen allergy have an allergy to fruits and vegetables. Note that the reaction occurs with raw fruit and vegetables; when they are cooked it is not usually present. It typically presents as tingling, itching and swelling in the oropharyngeal area but can also include urticaria, angioedema, wheeze and abdominal pain.

Causes

Patients suffering from allergic rhinitis caused by birch pollen (primarily an airborne allergen) may notice their mouth or throat becomes itchy after eating stone fruit, apple, carrot, peanuts, almond, hazelnuts or celery, mostly in the springtime. This reaction, called cross-reactivity, occurs because the proteins found in some fruits and vegetables are very similar to those found in birch pollen. These proteins can confuse the immune system and cause an allergic reaction, OAS, also called pollen fruit syndrome (PFS). These patients have a positive skin-prick test or blood test for birch pollen.

Similar effects can occur with grass pollen allergy, with the potential for cross-reactivity to peaches, celery, tomatoes, melons and oranges, and with ragweed allergy, in which the patient might have symptoms with banana, cucumber, melon, and courgette (zucchini).

Individuals who respond to cooked foods have more severe allergies.

Diagnosis

The history will help to identify the presence of OAS. Usually, people have seasonal allergic rhinitis before they develop OAS. This is because the proteins in the fruit, vegetables or nuts causing OAS are similar to those in the pollen causing the hay fever. Skin-prick testing can be useful in determining the exact cause, in conjunction with the history.

Management

The patient should avoid eating the trigger foods raw, especially during allergy season, because in many cases symptoms get worse during the pollen season. It is believed that cooking or baking the food at high temperatures breaks down the proteins responsible for the symptoms.

Peeling the skin off the food where possible, as the offending protein is often concentrated in the skin, and eating canned food may also elicit a smaller reaction.

Reactions to nuts need to be taken seriously, with specialist advice requested.

Individuals for whom the cooked food is not a problem can keep it in their diet. Otherwise, avoidance is very important. As this can mean a loss of sources of nutrients such as vitamins and minerals, patients should be educated about maintaining a balanced diet.

If the patient is at risk of severe reactions, then adrenaline auto-injectors can be considered. Antihistamines can be provided to be used if required.

3.8 Drug allergy

Drug reactions are not uncommon. These reactions are mostly diagnosed in specialist clinics in hospital, as medications are stopped in primary care if allergy is suspected. It is impossible to predict drug allergy.

Drug allergy can be IgE- and non-IgE-mediated. For example, penicillin allergy involves IgE-mediated mechanisms, whereas opiates, NSAIDs and contrast dye used in radiological imaging produce angioedema and anaphylaxis by non-IgE-mediated mechanisms.

In non-IgE-mediated conditions, the type IV cell-mediated mechanism can be involved. This type IV reaction was further subdivided into four types by WJ Pichler after his work on differentiating cellular mechanisms involved in drug hypersensitivity reactions.

Should an allergy be suspected, it is important to document the index drug, reaction including time of onset, and other medications being taken at that time. A drug allergy history can be challenging; NICE guidelines are available (2014, CG183) that provide information for documentation, the nature of patient drug allergy and a list of drugs to be avoided. British Society of Allergy and Clinical Immunology guidelines (2008, see www.bsaci.org/guidelines/drug-allergy) are also available to help clinicians. Management of drug allergy includes discontinuing the drug, providing antihistamines and referral to the allergist for confirmation and planning for future treatment. Anaphylactic reaction will need to be dealt with as described in *Section 3.1.1*.

3.8.1 Penicillin

This is one of the most well-known drug allergies. Penicillin allergy can present under any of the four hypersensitivity reactions.

Severe reactions are uncommon but anaphylaxis can occur with intravenous administration. There is approximately 8% cross-reactivity with cephalosporin antibiotics.

Avoidance is key, and alternative treatments should be prescribed as appropriate.

3.9 Latex allergy

Pure latex allergy presents as a type I hypersensitivity reaction. The type IV reactions that are sometimes seen are due to the plasticisers used in the manufacturing process.

Cross-reactions are common and include reactions to papaya, avocado, pineapple, bananas, lettuce, kiwi, potatoes and tomatoes.

Diagnosis

The history can be diagnostic; the use of skin-prick testing can provide additional help.

Management

Avoidance is key, so occupational health services should be contacted to advise the patient on how best to avoid the allergen depending on their situation, for example where they are most likely to be exposed to the allergen. Alternatives to latex should also be provided, if available.

Treatment for an anaphylactic response is described in *Section 3.1.1*.

3.10 Insect allergy

Insect allergies are common in summer. Their incidence varies in different parts of the country. Common culprits include bees and wasps, the sting of which can provoke a reaction, and biting insects, which in the UK include midges, mosquitoes, fleas, ticks and bed bugs. These reactions are not IgE-mediated but caused by enzymes, histamine, peptides, vasoactive amines and other mediators; the reaction is local in most cases (though commonly large in size), but does carry the risk of anaphylaxis. The most common venom allergies are to wasp and bee stings, which can cause severe reactions.

Diagnosis

A detailed history coupled with local and systemic examination is essential. The history can often indicate the source of the venom and the reaction that occurred.

Skin-prick testing can be useful, though it must be avoided if there is a history of anaphylaxis. Graded venom concentrations can be helpful, especially if the history is inconclusive as to the source of the venom.

Management

Avoidance is essential. Patients at risk of anaphylaxis should be given an adrenaline auto-injector kit with an appropriate action plan and training in its usage.

In severe cases, immunotherapy can be considered, if appropriate, by specialists with experience.

3.11 Others

3.11.1 Sulphite sensitivity

Some individuals can react to sulphite agents, found in foods and drinks as preservatives and antioxidants. Reactions may present as flushing, wheeziness or tachycardia, all the way through to an anaphylaxis-like reaction.

Causes

The cause of sulphite sensitivity remains unclear.

Diagnosis

Identifying the trigger through the history is of crucial importance. If required, a challenge test can be performed in a controlled setting with experts present.

Management

Avoidance is the mainstay of treatment and as such adequate advice must be given to patients. If indicated, adrenaline auto-injectors can be given for severe reactions.

3.11.2 Aspirin sensitivity

Aspirin sensitivity can present as a triad of asthma, nasal polyposis and rhinitis/rhinosinusitis, or as single symptoms of the triad. It can also be present with other NSAIDs presenting with angioedema.

Causes

Intolerance of cyclo-oxygenase 1 inhibition leads to a loss of bronchodilating prostaglandins and production of bronchoconstricting leukotrienes.

Diagnosis

The history will indicate a temporal relationship between the symptoms and use of a compound.

Management

Exclusion is the mainstay of treatment and so adequate education is important. Nasal polyps and sinusitis should be managed by ear, nose and throat specialists in appropriate secondary care settings.

Chapter 4

Asthma: background and clinical presentation

4.1	Pathophysiology	56
4.2	Risk factors for asthma	57
4.3	Stratification of asthma	57
4.4	Diagnosis	57
4.5	Differential diagnoses	60
4.6	Asthma attack	63
4.7	Complications of asthma	63

Asthma is a common respiratory disease, of the class of obstructive airways conditions, and can present acutely or with a chronic picture. It affects 5.4 million people in the UK and an estimated 300 million people worldwide, with a higher incidence in children than in adults. In early childhood, asthma is more common in boys, but by adulthood, the gender ratio is reversed.

Whilst the majority of asthma is due to atopy (approximately 80%), it is estimated that occupational asthma may account for up to 15% of adult-onset asthma.

Although asthma is recognised as a long-term condition that requires ongoing management, a significant proportion of children with asthma are seen to 'grow out' of it, or symptomatically improve over time. Nonetheless, it accounts for 2–3% of primary care presentations and approximately 60 000 hospital admissions per annum in the UK. It remains a deadly condition; over 1400 people died from asthma in the UK in 2016.

This section is based on the latest guidelines (2019) from the British Thoracic Society (BTS) and Scottish Intercollegiate Guideline Network (SIGN, 158).

4.1 Pathophysiology

Asthma results from a complex interplay between immune cells, mediator and structural airway cells leading to airway inflammation, bronchial hyper-responsiveness and reversible exaggerated airflow obstruction due to smooth muscle contraction. Interestingly, biopsies have shown that the key players in this inflammatory process are of the same nature as those seen in allergic reactions, irrespective of the atopy status of the patient.

The reaction itself is regarded as an early-phase bronchoconstriction following allergen exposure, followed by a late-phase recurrence.

In the acute phase, IgE cross-links with antigen, causing mast-cell degranulation (also includes basophils, eosinophils and macrophages) and release of mediators such as histamine, prostaglandin D2, cysteinyl leukotrienes and interleukins. It may also include neural pathway activation ultimately causing smooth muscle contraction, vasodilatation with subsequent oedema, and increased mucus secretion. A subgroup of asthmatics are non-eosinophilic and instead have neutrophil-mediated airway inflammation.

The late-phase reaction is led by the inflammatory cells that have permeated the airways during the early phase. It includes elements of the innate and adaptive immune responses, in particular the type 2 T helper cell immune responses.

Importantly, asthma can lead to irreversible changes. The recurrence of acute symptoms causes acute-on-chronic symptoms leading to airway remodelling, increased severity of symptoms and deterioration of lung function.

4.2 Risk factors for asthma

Asthma has a complex inheritance pattern, but research has not revealed specific genes or specific gene–environment interactions that cause asthma. However, some chromosomal regions have been found that are related to elements of the disease, that is, the production of IgE antibodies, airway hyper-responsiveness and the production of inflammatory mediators.

Those with a history of other atopic conditions (e.g. eczema or allergic rhinitis) are at increased risk of developing asthma. Other risk factors for early asthma development include maternal smoking, significant use of antibiotics within the first two years of life, being born preterm and delivery by caesarean section.

The discussion behind breastfeeding and the incidence of allergic disease is an extensive one. We will not cover it here, since as it stands evidence on the association with asthma is conflicting. The 'hygiene hypothesis' is also of interest and under investigation; however, it too has issues in its association with the pathogenesis of asthma.

Evidence links a high body mass index to asthma; however, the magnitude of the effect has not yet been proven.

Research in women during pregnancy has revealed evidence that a diet containing fish-oil-derived fatty acids, vitamin E and zinc plays a protective role against wheeze and asthma in young children.

4.3 Stratification of asthma

The asthma phenotype uses the observable characteristics of the patient's asthma – clinical and biological properties – to categorise the disease. The most common categories are:
* allergic asthma
* non-allergic asthma
* late-onset asthma
* asthma with fixed airflow limitation
* asthma with obesity.

Asthma endotypes are categorised by specific biological mechanisms and can encompass various phenotypes. This is an area of much current interest and research, with the aim of achieving effective, personalised treatments.

4.4 Diagnosis

There is no single diagnostic test to confirm asthma; it is a clinical diagnosis with objective supporting evidence. To diagnose this condition, the presence of suggestive symptoms must be demonstrated, along with airflow variability and airway hyper-responsiveness, all in the absence of an alternative explanation. This requires a detailed history (see *Section 4.4.1*). The timing of the symptoms as well as triggers of exacerbations can indicate the aetiology of the condition. It is important to identify factors that may increase the risk of asthma or trigger its symptoms:

- if patient is presenting outside of childhood, personal history of respiratory symptoms as a child
- birth history – whether born preterm
- personal and family history of atopy e.g. eczema, rhinitis, sinusitis, conjunctivitis, hay fever, nasal polyp, food allergies
- history of smoking or exposure to second-hand smoke (although this is not solely indicative)
- presence of household pets or carpeted areas
- history of exposure to irritants
- exclude alternative diagnoses (see *Section 4.5* for further details), including acute infection.

Symptomatic patients may present with a clinically urgent presentation in the form of an 'asthma attack'. Severity must be gauged accurately as it will determine further management, as described in *Chapter 5*.

The clinician should perform a complete examination of the respiratory system including recording basic observations such as the respiratory rate, heart rate and blood pressure (though this may be challenging in children, so should be done opportunistically during the assessment). Because asthma findings have significant variability, the absence of physical findings does not exclude a diagnosis of asthma. Generally, a positive examination may reveal a prolonged expiratory phase or an expiratory wheeze on auscultation of the chest, denoting airflow limitation.

The physical examination should also include examination of the skin for signs of other atopic conditions, close inspection of the eyes and examination of the upper respiratory tract including nose, throat and pharynx.

4.4.1 Symptoms

The classical symptoms are:
- recurrent and episodic wheeze
- chest tightness
- shortness of breath
- persistent cough
- excessive mucus production.

Note that there is usually more than one respiratory symptom. They are often variable over time; usually worst at night/on waking and made worse during an infection. Episodes vary in intensity and frequency, sometimes self-terminating, other times needing treatment. Patients may go weeks or months without symptoms.

Identifying triggers is vital; specific triggers could be related to the allergy itself, whether seasonal or perennial (e.g. pollens and cat and dog dander, respectively), or be non-specific (e.g. exercise, cold air, perfumes, medications – NSAIDs or beta-blockers – and even laughter). Note there may be exercise limitation.

Occupational asthma can occur in, but not limited to, laboratory workers, bakers, animal handlers, welders, paint industry workers, wood workers, gardeners and builders. Their symptoms improve at the weekend or when on holiday. These patients should be referred to a specialist.

4.4.2 Airflow variability and obstruction

This can be objectively evidenced by carrying out twice-daily peak flow readings (repeat readings can be done when patients feel symptomatic) over a two-week period. It is important that the same peak flow meter is used and optimal technique is confirmed to ensure accurate readings. The best of three readings should be recorded each time. A variation of more than 20% is indicative of asthma. The more occasions on which such variation is demonstrated, the greater the confidence in the diagnosis can be.

Features of asthma on spirometry with bronchodilator reversibility test include:
- a reduced FEV_1
- a reduced FEV_1/FVC ratio (normally >0.75–0.80 in adults, >0.90 in children)
- bronchodilator reversibility of >12% FEV_1 or >200 ml from baseline 10–15 minutes after bronchodilator (>13% in children).

A normal spirometry result in asymptomatic individuals does not exclude asthma.

The FeNO test is becoming increasingly available in secondary care and can be helpful for diagnosis in both adults and children with an intermediate probability of asthma yet normal spirometry (without challenge testing). If elevated, it may indicate eosinophilic inflammation, supporting a diagnosis of asthma. However, a negative test does not rule asthma out. There are still issues with the test; exhaled nitric oxide can be elevated in patients with allergic rhinitis, in men and following dietary consumption of nitrates, whereas it can be reduced in smokers and in those using steroids. Also, it may not be raised in asthma phenotypes with neutrophilic inflammation.

4.5 Differential diagnoses

As there is no single definitive test to diagnose asthma it is important that a complete history is taken to explore for alternative diagnoses. For example, a cough as the only presenting respiratory symptom in adults is unlikely to be asthma (there is a cough-variant asthma, but other causes of cough must first be excluded), and the history should be used to explore for the possibility of drug-induced cough (e.g. ACE inhibitor use), gastroesophageal reflux disease, post-nasal drip and so on. Possible differential diagnoses for asthma and key distinguishing factors are considered in *Tables 4.1* and *4.2* from a disease-focused point of view.

Where it is difficult to establish the diagnosis of asthma or alternative diagnoses are plausible (especially if there are red flag features) then patients should be referred to a specialist.

Table 4.1 Differential diagnosis for asthma originating in respiratory tract pathology. GI, gastrointestinal.

*Hyperinflated state can be indicated by a reduced cricosternal distance with protuberant abdomen.

**COPD can be a separate entity or part of an overlap syndrome with asthma.

	Chest tightness	Dyspnoea	Cough	Sputum	Wheeze	Clinical examination
Bronchiectasis Chest infections as a child, recurrent exposure to smoke or biofuels	+/−	++	+++	+++	++	May have clubbing or be cyanosed ++ Inspiratory coarse crackles Occasional clicks and squeaks
Cystic fibrosis Presenting from childhood, cause of bronchiectasis Multisystem disease including GI symptoms	−	+/−	+++	+	−	Short stature and thin with clubbing As above
COPD** Recurrent infective exacerbation Exposure to smoke Not clubbed	+/−	++ Exertional	+++	++	+++	Pursed-lipped breathing and hyperinflated* Hyper-resonant on percussion with expiratory wheeze and coarse inspiratory crackles
Foreign body Risk factors e.g. in children or mental illness	−	−	Sudden onset, persistent	−	+ Unilateral or stridor (foreign body location)	Sudden onset (seconds) Reduced chest movement on affected side Reduced breath sounds distal to obstruction

Table 4.2 Differential diagnosis for asthma originating in pathology in other systems or processes. PND, paroxysmal nocturnal dyspnoea.

	Chest pain	Dyspnoea	Cough	Sputum	Wheeze	Notes
Pulmonary embolism	+ Pleuritic	++ Acute onset	+ Haemoptysis	–	–	Examination may be normal or evidence of secondary pleural effusion. ECG is important. Risk factor assessment is key
Dysfunctional breathing	Variable May be tightness	Variable Hyperventilation Sighing	Variable	–	–	May make wheeze-like sounds that are actually from upper airway Present episodically, associated with dizziness/light-headedness, peripheral tingling
Gastro-oesophageal reflux	May be described as burning	+	+	–	+/–	Postural and food-related symptoms. May be associated with voice changes, soreness in throat or retching
Left ventricle dysfunction	Unless acute event	+ On exertion When severe, at rest	+ If in pulmonary oedema			Peripheral oedema may be present Nocturnal symptoms: orthopnoea and PND History of cardiac disease
Vocal cord dysfunction		+			Stridor	History is usually diagnostic.

4.6 Asthma attack

Patients may present with acute or subacute symptoms that need to be assessed for severity (*Table 4.3*), which will determine treatment and the best place for management. Anyone with signs of life-threatening/severe asthma attack or a history of previous near-fatal asthma should be managed in hospital. This decision is patient-specific: there may be other reasons why someone with a moderate asthma attack needs to be reviewed in hospital (e.g. recent severe attack or nocturnal symptoms, concerns over social circumstance).

Table 4.3 Categorisation of severity of asthma attacks.

Category / Variable	Moderate	Acute severe	Life-threatening
Bedside inspection	Talks in full sentences	Cannot complete full sentence in one breath	Exhausted, cyanotic, altered consciousness
Respiratory rate per minute	<25	≥25 (5–12 years old >30, 2–5 years old >40)	Poor respiratory effort
Heart rate per minute	<110	≥110 (5–12 years old >125, 2–5 years old >140)	≥110 or arrythmia
Clinical examination	Wheeze +/– infection	Wheeze ++ +/– infection	Hypotension Silent chest
Peak flow % of best or predicted	>50–75%	33–55%	<33%
Oxygen saturations	≥92%	≥92%	<92%
Arterial blood gas			Acidaemia CO_2 within normal range or rising ($PaCO_2$ >4.6 kPa) Hypoxia, taking into account the inspired oxygen concentration

Those with acute severe or life-threatening asthma who do not respond to therapy and those requiring ventilatory support should be referred to the intensive therapy unit (ITU). Principles of management can be found in the next section.

It is always important to try to identify the trigger for the attack; allergen exposure and infection are amongst the commonest causes.

4.7 Complications of asthma

If asthma is not adequately controlled then patients may suffer from repeated asthma attacks, pneumothorax, lung collapse, pneumonia and ultimately respiratory failure. In the long term, irreversible structural changes occur in the parenchyma and musculature.

Asthma can also have a detrimental impact on the patient's psychological wellbeing, implications for education and work (due to sick leave and fatigue), and the poor sleep and exercise intolerance can lead to metabolic complications, hypertension and obesity.

Chapter 5

Asthma: management

5.1   Acute asthma management   66

5.2   Chronic asthma management   67

5.3   Monitoring asthma   73

5.4   Paediatric asthma   74

Asthma is a common chronic inflammatory condition; patient empowerment, insight and engagement lie at the heart of its management, along with an up-to-date personalised action plan based on the patient's current clinical state. Clinicians should aim to prevent daytime symptoms, to stop night-time awakening due to asthma and reduce to nil usage of the reliever inhaler (i.e. short-acting beta-2 agonist). Together, the clinician and patient should work together to maintain control on the minimum possible dose of medicine.

Asthma symptom control can be achieved through pharmacological therapies and avoidance of trigger factors. To ensure medication is targeted to the respiratory tract, it is delivered through an inhaler, with a variety of devices available on the market. Inhaler technique is crucial, hence time should be spent on demonstrating and then assessing it, as well as providing resources that patients can later return to (poor technique even after training is not uncommon). Patients should receive counselling on how to use the medication, and on the side-effects and how to prevent them (e.g. rinsing the mouth after using inhaled corticosteroid).

There are two principal types of inhalers available: pressurised metered-dose inhaler (MDI) and dry powder inhaler (DPI). Not all medications are available in every delivery device. Some devices have dose counters.

Spacers are plastic devices with a mouthpiece at one end and a hole for a pressurised MDI to be inserted at the other end. A spacer with face mask is recommended for children (2–4 years of age). Its main purpose is to increase the drug delivery to the lining of the airways. Spacers should be regularly washed and allowed to air-dry, and replaced according to the manufacturer's advice.

There are different types of medications available to minimise asthma symptoms:
- relievers (short-acting beta-2 agonists)
- preventers (inhaled corticosteroids)
- add-on therapies (long-acting beta-2 agonist, leukotriene receptor antagonist, theophylline, long-acting muscarinic antagonist).

Medical therapy varies according to asthma severity, asthma control and the age of the patient.

5.1 Acute asthma management

In the first instance, severity of the exacerbation must be gauged (see *Section 4.6, Asthma attack*).

5.1.1 In the community

If the patient has an asthma attack of moderate severity (see *Section 4.6*) then begin with a short-acting beta-2 agonist therapy (usually nebulised through oxygen).

This should be combined with a dose of steroid: prednisolone can be given orally, or intravenous hydrocortisone is also available. Give supplemental oxygen to maintain saturations of 94–98%.

If the attack is severe and the patient has not responded to treatment, they should be admitted to hospital. Patients with asthma attacks classified as life-threatening should go to the hospital straight away irrespective of response to treatment.

5.1.2 In-hospital management

The step-by-step detailed approach for in-hospital care goes beyond the scope of this book, but a basic outline is given below.

Severe asthma attacks require nebulised short-acting beta-2 agonist (can be used very frequently; in life-threatening attacks, it can be used every 15–30 minutes) along with nebulised short-acting muscarinic antagonist (maximum four times a day), supplemental oxygen to keep saturation at 94–98% and a dose of steroids (oral prednisolone or intravenous hydrocortisone).

A chest radiograph should be requested to look for signs of consolidation or pneumothorax. Blood tests including blood gases should also be considered; the latter to help assess the severity of the exacerbation. Life-threatening features should be identified straight away, as these patients need senior medical and ITU review. They may also need intravenous therapies such as magnesium sulphate or aminophylline. They may even require mechanical ventilation.

5.2 Chronic asthma management

The latest British Thoracic Society/Scottish Intercollegiate Guidelines Network (BTS/SIGN) guidelines on asthma management advocate the treatment regime shown in *Figure 5.1*.

The following section should provide an understanding of drugs used in the management of asthma. Please refer to the BNF (or your national formulary) and/or Trust guidelines for recommended drugs, doses, side-effects and drug interactions.

5.2.1 Beta-2 agonists: short-acting

Short-acting beta-2 agonists (SABAs) are the main reliever medication. Asthmatic patients should be prescribed one. It stimulates the beta-2 adrenergic receptor found in the smooth muscle lining the airways, causing the muscle to relax and consequently dilating the airway. SABAs are available in a variety of forms: tablet, syrup, inhaler and for nebulised use (the last used in acute asthma to turn the liquid form into a fine mist once nebulised, allowing inhalation of a large dose

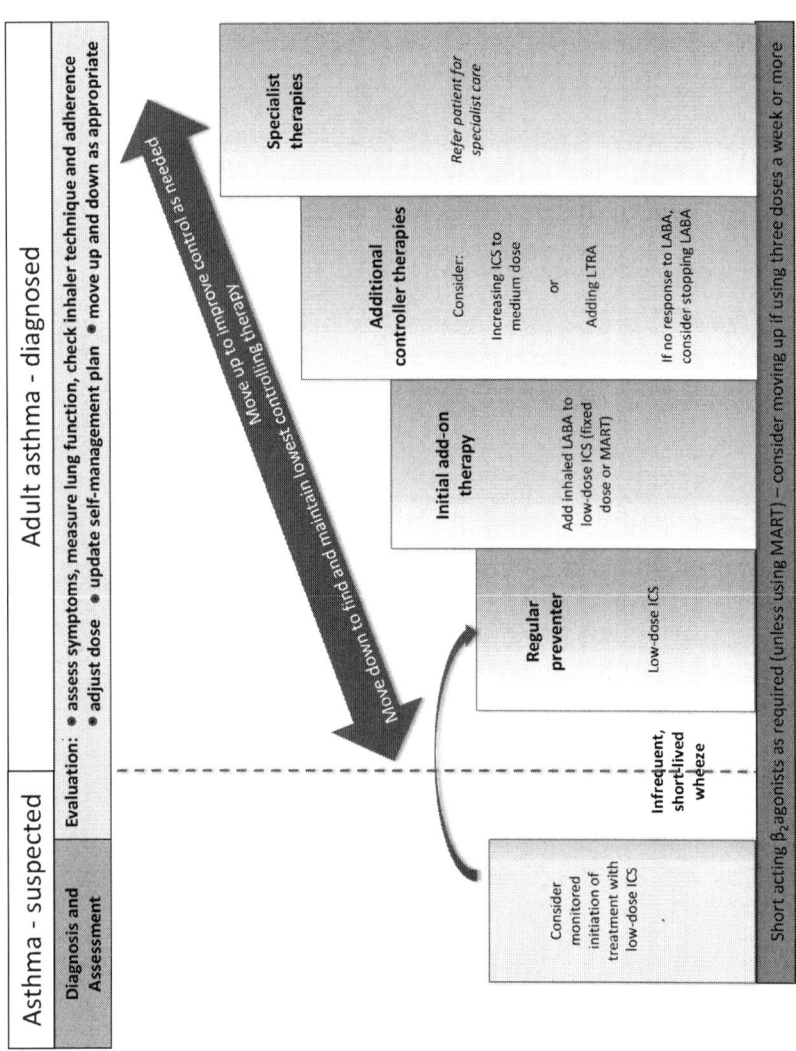

Figure 5.1 Summary of management of asthma in adults, reproduced from BTS/SIGN British Guideline on the Management of Asthma 2019 with permission. ICS, inhaled corticosteroid; LABA, long-acting beta-2 agonist; LTRA, leukotriene receptor antagonist; MART, maintenance and reliever therapy.

of the medicine). It has a rapid onset of action, approximately 15 minutes, and its effect lasts for up to 4 hours. Commonly used preparations are salbutamol and terbutaline.

In a small minority of people with infrequent, short-lived wheeze (which may be seasonal) and normal lung function, this may be the only medication required. The treatment regime is considered inadequate if symptoms are not fully relieved by this treatment or if a SABA is required more than three times a week (not necessarily during a viral respiratory infection).

Patients who develop asthma symptoms as a result of predictable triggers like exercise-induced bronchoconstriction and exposure to cold air are encouraged to use their SABA approximately 10 to 20 minutes before exposure or exercise in order to prevent the development of symptoms.

5.2.2 Beta-2 agonists: long-acting

Long-acting beta-2 agonist (LABA) monotherapy is not recommended for patients with asthma as it does not affect airway inflammation and is associated with an increased risk of morbidity and mortality. It is advised only in combination with inhaled corticosteroids (ICSs). The combination of a LABA and ICS has shown to be highly effective in reducing asthma symptoms and exacerbations.

It is a preferred treatment option in adolescents or adults whose asthma is inadequately controlled on low-dose ICS therapy, or in children over 6 years of age whose asthma is uncontrolled on moderate ICS doses. This medicine should be introduced at a low dose initially and the effect should be monitored for 4 weeks before considering a dose alteration.

LABA duration of action is 12 hours. Its adverse effects are similar to that of SABA. They are usually dose-related, and include: fine tremor in hands, worse in the first few days of treatment; hypokalaemia, palpitations, headache, anxiety, dizziness, cardiac arrhythmias and acute angle-closure glaucoma. Rarely bronchospasm or seizure can occur. They should be used with caution in patients with hyperthyroidism, diabetes mellitus, hypertension or cardiovascular disease.

5.2.3 Corticosteroids: inhaled

ICS is known as 'preventer' medication. It is the mainstay of treatment for adults and children suffering from asthma as it reduces airway inflammation, bronchial hyper-responsiveness, improves quality of life and decreases the risk of serious exacerbations of asthma.

The dose should be based on the severity of disease and the patient's age. The lowest possible dose to achieve optimal control should be used. The patient should be reviewed after 4 weeks, and the dose can be increased if their asthma is not controlled. Once good control is established, the same daily dose can be considered as maintenance therapy.

Smoking reduces the effectiveness of ICS therapy, therefore current or ex-smokers may need higher doses of ICS.

If ICS therapy is unsuccessful in achieving asthma control, the clinician should look for factors such as poor adherence, improper inhaler technique, continued exposure to a trigger and misdiagnosis of the disease. Ultimately, if steroids remain an appropriate option, treatment should be modified by stepping up to a high dose or to the next therapy, which may even mean oral steroids.

Common side-effects with ICS therapy are oropharyngeal candidiasis and dysphonia (hoarseness of voice). Rinsing the mouth with water after each treatment and the use of a spacer with MDI devices can help to reduce the risk of these side-effects. Systemic adverse effects of steroids from ICS therapy are rare but may occur at high doses, especially in children. They include decreased bone density, cataract, glaucoma, growth failure in children and signs of adrenal suppression.

5.2.4 Corticosteroids: oral

Oral corticosteroids, usually in the form of prednisolone, are used in the management regime for acute exacerbation of asthma (as a short course) and for maintenance therapy in people with chronic uncontrolled asthma (under the care of a specialist).

The prolonged use of oral steroids is associated with well-known and serious adverse effects. Therefore their routine or long-term use should be avoided, particularly in children. Adverse events with short-term, high-dose oral prednisolone can cause reversible change in glucose metabolism, polyphagia and weight gain (though this can also be due to fluid retention) and hypertension.

Patients should be given a steroid treatment card during their treatment. A patient using steroid tablets for longer than 3 months should be monitored for adrenal suppression, have regular blood pressure and blood sugar checks, be monitored for bone mineral density (to identify signs of osteoporosis), have regular vision checks for cataracts and glaucoma, and growth checks in children in case of growth retardation.

5.2.5 Leukotriene receptor antagonists

The most commonly used leukotriene receptor antagonist (LTRA) is montelukast. LTRAs are an oral therapy, taken at night as an add-on to a combination of ICS and LABA. LTRAs used as monotherapy are less effective than ICS treatment.

Leukotrienes are produced in response to mast-cell degranulation during an allergic reaction. Thus LTRAs help to ease both allergy and asthma symptoms. They also decrease the number of activated eosinophils present in inflamed mucosa, and are helpful for symptoms of rhinorrhoea and nasal congestion. LTRAs can be prescribed for patients from the age of 5 years onward.

The duration of the add-on treatment depends on the response of the patient to treatment: ideally, the prevention of daytime symptoms, nocturnal awakening and asthma attacks, and improved quality of life. Once a person's asthma has been controlled with their current maintenance therapy for at least 3 months, consider decreasing the maintenance therapy. Reductions in asthma treatment should be carried out slowly and under close observation, as every patient responds differently to the reduction. It is recommended to decrease the dose by 25% every 3 months and follow up to check the response.

These medications may have significant adverse effects in some patients, so regular follow-up and advice to the patient is recommended. Patients should be advised to seek medical advice urgently if they observe any psychological symptoms. A very small percentage of patients may develop eosinophilic granulomatosis with polyangiitis (Churg–Strauss syndrome), which is characterised by systemic eosinophilia, eosinophilic pneumonia, vasculitis and arthritis.

5.2.6 Anticholinergics

Muscarinic antagonists work by blocking the cholinergic nerves that release mediators causing constriction of the muscles lining the airway. The short-acting form, commonly ipratropium bromide, is used to treat acute exacerbation. It has a slower onset of action, approximately 20 minutes, and achieves significantly less bronchodilation in asthma than inhaled SABAs.

A long-acting form, tiotropium bromide, is commonly used as an add-on therapy in combination with ICS and LABA. It improves lung function and in some cases protects against acute asthma exacerbations.

5.2.7 Theophylline

An add-on therapy, theophylline works by relaxing the smooth muscles of the bronchial airway and pulmonary blood vessels to reduce airway response to histamine. The medication has a significant side-effect profile and should be started under the advice and supervision of an asthma specialist. Regular blood checks, including measuring the serum level of theophylline, are necessary. Oral medicine does not help in acute attacks; in such cases intravenous preparations are used.

5.2.8 Cromones

Cromones are used as an add-on therapy. They work by inhibiting the release of inflammatory mediators, especially from lung mast cells, in response to airway irritation. Ultimately they stabilise mast cells and decrease inflammation. Cromones have been shown to be beneficial in adults and children older than 5 years.

The commonly used drugs are sodium cromoglicate and nedocromil sodium. Cromones have almost no systemic absorption and negligible systemic adverse effects; their only common side-effects are transient cough due to direct irritation by the powder through use of an inhaler or transient stinging in eyes when used as an eye-drop preparation. This medication should be discontinued if the patient develops eosinophilic pneumonia. It can also cause a paradoxical bronchospasm (though frequency is not known). If this occurs, treatment with cromones should be discontinued.

5.2.9 Bronchial thermoplasty

This invasive procedure works by reducing smooth muscle bulk by treating the airways with a series of radiofrequency pulses. It reduces the frequency of severe asthma exacerbations and improves quality of life.

Bronchial thermoplasty is not a common management tool in asthma. It can be considered for adult patients with severe asthma that is not under control despite optimal pharmacotherapy. Even then, the assessment should be done by an asthma specialist with expertise in bronchial thermoplasty, and the patient should be listed on the UK Severe Asthma Registry. This treatment may only be carried out in specialist centres. It requires long-term follow-up.

5.2.10 Immunomodulatory therapy

Immunomodulatory therapy is a potentially disease-modifying treatment for allergy and asthma patients; it has already been successful in allergic rhinitis. It is not the first-line treatment for allergic asthma and should be used only with the supervision and advice of an immunologist and asthma specialist.

Immunotherapy involves regular administration of a tiny dose of the allergen, usually subcutaneous or sublingual. In this process, the dose administered is gradually increased until it is effective at inducing immunologic tolerance to the allergen. Through this treatment the patient's immune system builds up a tolerance to the allergen over time, and the allergic reaction diminishes. This treatment generally requires regular therapy (varies based on the medication itself, ranging from daily treatment to treatment only taken for a few months in the year) over a period of 3–5 years with regular follow-up.

5.2.11 Advances in asthma treatment

New asthma treatments work at a cellular level by blocking the role of IgE in the steps leading to allergic asthma. One example is omalizumab injections, the treatment of choice for moderate to severe persistent allergic asthma in patients over 6 years of age who have a high steroid burden and who meet the serological criteria.

5.3 Monitoring asthma

New diagnoses of asthma should be reviewed regularly (e.g. every 6 months). In addition, some cases should be monitored more closely, including patients with a history of an asthma attack within the last 3 months that had to be treated with oral corticosteroid, or of repeated flare-ups in spite of treatment. More regular follow-up is required in people undergoing treatment adjustment and patients with psychosocial problems and non-concordance to treatment. With new patients, it is important to explore any sign or symptoms of anxiety or depression as these are more common in people with asthma.

In general, for all patients under follow-up in primary care, it is important to monitor regularly for:
- symptom control (details below) and asthma attack history
- lung function (using spirometry or by peak expiratory flow rates)
- social implications including time off work.

Medication review focuses on checking:
- inhaler technique
- frequency of rescue inhaler use and concordance with inhaled therapies (including any side-effects)
- frequency of steroid use.

A personalised action plan reflective of the latest clinical status should always be available and the patient should possess a copy. This is in addition to any concerns the patient may have.

Symptom control can be gauged by checking whether the patient:

- is suffering from nocturnal symptoms
- is suffering from daytime symptoms
- finds that asthma has interfered with their activities.

It is important that patients can recognise deterioration in their symptoms and know where to seek medical advice if this happens. The same is true if contact with asthma triggers is unavoidable (though the clinician and patient should work together to try and reduce exposure to triggers as much as possible) – for example upper respiratory tract illnesses, physical exertion, hormonal fluctuations or extreme emotion. It may be of life-saving importance to ensure the patient has a reliever close at all times and knows where to seek help.

It is also good practice to check whether the patient's vaccinations are up to date (whether this be the childhood immunisations schedule or annual influenza vaccination in adults) and always check their smoking status (including exposure to second-hand smoke).

When assessing children, it is important to regularly check the child's growth (height and weight measurements) and mental development. There are validated questionnaires available (see BTS/SIGN guidelines 2019) to assess asthma control in children; there is also a questionnaire available for wheezy children who are at risk of developing asthma.

5.4 Paediatric asthma

This section focuses on the unique elements of paediatric asthma that have not already been covered.

Evaluation of children can be challenging for a number of reasons: young children may have difficulty expressing symptoms, there is significant overlap in symptomatology with that of acute infection (and frequency of infections) and formal assessment of lung function in young children is difficult. Triggers of asthma can vary depending on the age of the patient; in very young children the trigger is usually a viral infection, but food allergy is another possible cause.

In children with asthma, three wheeze phenotypes have been identified (*Table 5.1*).

Table 5.1 Wheeze phenotypes in children with asthma.

Transient early wheezing	Non-atopic wheezing	IgE-mediated atopic wheezing
• Symptoms limited to 3–5 years of age • Not associated with allergic sensitisation • Risk factors include reduced lung function diagnosed before any respiratory illness and maternal smoking during pregnancy.	• Symptoms begin in the first three years of life up until adolescence • Wheezing especially associated with viral infections • Milder phenotype than atopic phenotype.	• Persistent wheezing • Typified by early allergic sensitisation and airway hyper-responsiveness • Significant loss of lung function in early years of life.

5.4.1 Management of chronic asthma in children

In children under the age of 5 years who are unable to perform available tests, the clinician should use the history, clinical assessment and any positive objective result to help diagnose asthma. A useful method of confirming the diagnosis in young children is a trial of treatment.

The latest British Thoracic Society guidelines on asthma management for children advocate the treatment regime shown in *Figure 5.2*. It is also recommended that children receiving daily ICS therapy do not increase their daily ICS dose with the onset of a viral illness.

Optimal medication delivery by device and correct technique is important. In children, use a pMDI and spacer; a spacer with facemask is recommended for children 4–6 years of age or if the child is unable to tolerate a spacer with a mouthpiece. In adolescence preference should be taken into account regarding the choice of pMDI or DPI in order to optimise concordance with the medication. A DPI is generally not recommended for children under 6 years old given that the child must have sufficient inspiratory force to use it effectively.

Children with exercise-induced asthma should use their asthma preventer inhaler 15–20 minutes before physical exercise. A child with dust allergy should have well ventilated classrooms and be supported in avoiding exposure to dust from materials (clothing, chalk) which may generate it.

Optimal asthma management requires a multidisciplinary team approach, which includes the school nurse and teachers. They should be aware of the diagnosis, triggers and treatment plan including management of an emergency. The child should have easy access to their treatment, which the key staff members should know how to use.

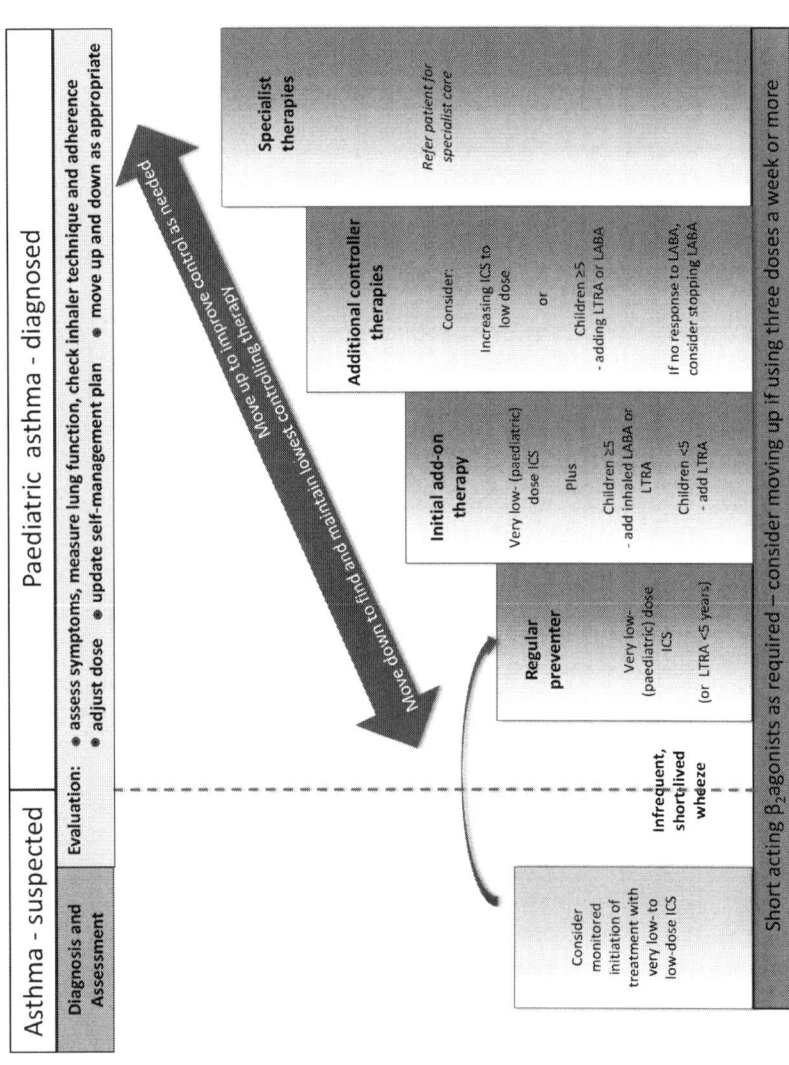

Figure 5.2 Summary of management of asthma in children, reproduced from the BTS/SIGN British Guideline on the Management of Asthma 2019, with permission. ICS, inhaled corticosteroid; LABA, long-acting beta-2 agonist; LTRA, leukotriene receptor antagonist.

Chapter 6
Management principles in allergy

6.1   Pharmacotherapy   78

Allergy is a common condition with significant associated morbidity, and in severe cases mortality. It often requires a multidisciplinary team approach, for example from primary care physicians, allergists, otorhinolaryngologists, ophthalmologists, respiratory physicians, paediatricians, dermatologists and immunologists.

One of the best treatments for allergy remains avoidance of the precipitating allergen. However, this is not always possible, and so patients suffering from allergies may need pharmacotherapy to alleviate symptoms and improve their quality of life. Medications commonly prescribed include antihistamines and topical corticosteroids. In a large number of patients there is no single medical therapy that is effective and so combination therapies are advised.

For anaphylaxis, the treatment algorithm is explained in *Section 3.1.1*.

Immunotherapy is emerging as a disease-modifying treatment, but is still awaiting evidence and licencing for more widespread use.

6.1 Pharmacotherapy

Before administering any drug for the first time, it is important that the prescribing clinician takes a drug history (risk of drug interactions), identifies any previous intolerances or drug allergies (will influence choice of treatment) and notes whether the patient is pregnant or has renal or liver impairment (may affect the dosing). Patients should be appropriately counselled for use of the medication by the prescribing clinicians.

Each section below lists commonly used medication in that class; however, this is not an exhaustive list.

6.1.1 Antihistamines

The term 'antihistamines' usually refers to medications that block histamine-1 receptors (blockage of histamine-2 receptors is not clinically fully understood; it may be helpful in a small subgroup of allergic patients). Mast-cell stabilisers work by preventing the release of histamine (covered separately below).

First-generation (sedating) antihistamines prevent histamine release and help control symptoms. Newer (non-sedating) antihistamines act by competing with histamine at the receptor level with downstream action on inflammatory mediators and the inflammatory process. In cases that are difficult to control, a combination of sedating and non-sedating antihistamines can be used.

Antihistamines reduce excessive mucus formation and are significantly effective at reducing itching and sneezing. However, they are not effective on the symptom of nasal obstruction.

Clinicians should be aware of drug interactions with anticonvulsants, monoamine oxidase inhibitors and central nervous system depressants such as opiates.

Route

Oral or topical – nasal sprays and eye drops.

Commonly used medications

Antihistamine$_1$ (non-sedating):
- cetirizine
- loratidine
- fexofenadine.

Antihistamine$_1$ (sedating):
- chlorphenamine
- hydroxyzine
- ketotifen.

Antihistamine$_2$:
- cimetidine
- ranitidine.

Side-effect profile

Sedation is more common with first-generation antihistamines; however, as a caveat, non-sedating antihistamines too can be sedating when given in high doses in some patients.

Older medication can be associated with anticholinergic side-effects such as dry mouth and bladder neck obstruction (beware in particular in older male patients: risk of urinary retention). Increased intraocular pressure, weight gain or hair loss are also recognised side-effects.

Newer antihistamines are more cardioselective, hence there is a risk of cardiac arrhythmias when given with systemic antifungal medications, erythromycin, clarithromycin, quinine and grapefruit.

6.1.2 Mast-cell stabilisers

These drugs work by preventing degranulation of mast cells, hence must be given before mast-cell priming by the antigen/IgE (therefore, clinically results are achieved if used before an anticipated antigen exposure; the drug would not be helpful if used after mast-cell degranulation has occurred).

These medications are significantly helpful for nasal symptoms. They are probably one of the best treatments for allergic rhinitis in pregnant patients, as long as adherence and technique are maintained.

Route

Topical – nasal sprays, eye drops; subcutaneous.

Commonly used medications

Olopatadine (antihistamine and mast-cell stabilising activity, topical); mepolizumab and omalizumab (monoclonal antibody for IgE, subcutaneous).

6.1.3 Decongestants

This group of medications are vasoconstrictors or sympathomimetics. The mechanism of action is alpha-adrenergic stimulation or constriction of the arterioles supplying the soft tissue of the organ, which leads to diminution in pooled volume within the turbinates in the nose. This in turn leads to decongestion and relief of obstruction; however, the action is short-lived.

This group of medications should be avoided in allergic rhinitis, as nasal blockage is a recurrent feature. They are not recommended in children under 3 months of age.

These drugs interact with tricyclic antidepressants, monoamine oxidase inhibitors, some antihypertensives and central nervous system stimulants.

There are treatments available that combine decongestant with antihistamine for alleviation of nasal and sinus symptoms. Use of these combination treatments should be recommended only for short lengths of time.

Route

Topical – eye drops, nasal spray; oral; inhaled.

Commonly used medications

Xylometazoline, ephedrine, oxymetazoline.

Side-effect profile

Rebound nasal obstruction is important to recognise in heavy or long-term use; in most cases patients start taking a decongestant without realising this potential side-effect, termed rhinitis medicamentosa.

Other side-effects include anorexia and cardiovascular and central nervous system stimulation.

6.1.4 Corticosteroids

Corticosteroids do not prevent allergic reactions but reduce the swelling caused by the chemical mediators released in allergic reaction. They have multiple anti-inflammatory effects and work in both early- and late-phase reactions, mainly by decreasing capillary permeability and inhibiting inflammatory mediator synthesis (amongst other actions).

They have wide-reaching therapeutic impacts in disease of both the upper (particularly helpful in rhinorrhoea and nasal congestion) and lower respiratory tract, as well as in the allergy emergency of anaphylaxis and in skin lesions.

There are significant considerations for long-term steroid use, including side-effects (as below) and sick day rules.

Route of therapy

Oral; intravenous; inhaled; nasal sprays/drops; topical.

Commonly used medications

Multiple available: prednisolone (oral), hydrocortisone (intravenous), mometasone (nasal spray), budesonide (inhaled), fluticasone (nasal spray and inhaler).

Side-effect profile

Long-term steroids can reduce the physiological activity of the hypothalamic–pituitary–adrenal axis; therefore abruptly stopping exogenous steroids is associated with a risk of precipitating an Addisonian crisis.

Steroids can have the systemic side-effects shown in *Figure 6.1*. In addition, local side-effects to ICSs include nasal crusting, irritation and bleeding.

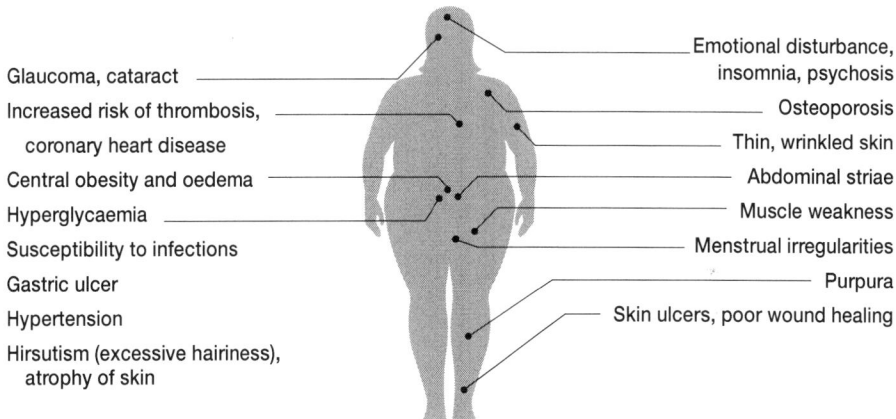

Figure 6.1 Systemic side-effects of steroid use, especially long-term.

Given the wide-ranging side-effects of steroids, drug history is of paramount importance. In particular, note that other drugs can exacerbate some of the side-effects of steroids; for example the concomitant use of NSAIDs (the risk of peptic ulcers), anticoagulants (the risk of bleeding) and digoxin (the risk of hypokalaemia when using corticosteroids and the consequent risk of increased digoxin toxicity).

6.1.5 Anticholinergics

Anticholinergic medications block the effects of acetylcholine on the muscarinic receptors, part of the parasympathetic nervous system. In the upper respiratory tract, these drugs are used to relieve rhinorrhoea (e.g. in vasomotor or allergic rhinitis) as they inhibit production of nasal mucus. In the lower respiratory tract, they work as bronchodilators (used in both acute and chronic presentations of asthma).

They can also be used, in different preparations, for neurological, gastrointestinal and genitourinary conditions.

Route

Topical – nasal drop, eye drops; inhaled; nebulised; oral.

Commonly used medications

Ipratropium bromide, tiotropium bromide (other preparations are available for non-respiratory tract indications).

Side-effect profile

Newer forms of the medications have fewer of the recognised side-effects of dry mouth, blurred vision, constipation and urinary retention.

Usually, especially when anticholinergics are used topically, side-effects are minimal, and long-term use does not lead to significant complications if used according to the advice of the clinician.

6.1.6 Leukotriene receptor antagonists

For full details, please see *Section 5.2.5*.

6.1.7 Immunotherapy

Immunotherapy is specialist treatment and should only be carried out in allergy centres; its current indications are allergic asthma, allergic rhinitis and food allergies. The aim is to achieve tolerance upon allergen exposure. Whilst the full pathway is yet to be understood, it is recognised that multiple cell types are affected, with end organs also showing changes that contribute to the overall tolerance observed. Put simply, mast-cell degranulation is reduced, antibody isotypes change (despite an early rise in IgE which later decreases, there is also a recognised consistent increase in allergen-specific IgG), allergen-specific T-regulatory and B-regulatory cells are generated (one of whose multiple functions is expression of various suppressor factors) and tissue mast cells and eosinophils decrease, amongst many other actions and changes.

Immunotherapy usually consists of a series of doses of varying dilutions of the causative allergens over months or years.

Route

Subcutaneous; sublingual.

Side-effect profile

Resuscitation equipment must be available at centres that carry out this procedure, as there is a risk of anaphylaxis. Local side-effects are fairly common, depending on the route of administration. However, as this is the latest, potentially curative, therapy whose specialist indications and use are constantly being updated, going into detail about side-effects goes beyond the scope of this book.

Chapter 7

Organ-specific treatment

7.1	Skin	86
7.2	Nose and sinuses	86
7.3	Ear	88
7.4	Eye	89
7.5	Chest and abdomen	89

This chapter brings together management principles for conditions classified by organ involved. Individual diseases can be found in the relevant section in *Chapter* 3.

Local, national and speciality-specific guidelines can be helpful, as they can guide management in a stepwise manner and also dictate the preferred therapy for patients.

7.1 Skin

Abnormal functioning of the affected area of skin can lead to onset of symptoms such as dryness, itching, redness, blistering or pigmentation, which can progressively worsen.

Key in the history is symptom onset, progression, response to previous treatment or recurrence, and the relationship between symptoms and exposures to possible triggers such as food and drinks, cosmetics, sunlight, animals, chemicals, latex and rubber. A detailed local and systemic examination should be carried out with appropriate investigations according to the circumstances of the disease.

It is important to remember the significant relationship between the skin and self-esteem and confidence. The psychological impact of skin diseases should not be underestimated; they can, for some, be socially isolating and debilitating, therefore professional input should be sought when needed.

Treatment of skin allergies starts with avoidance of the allergen. Topical moisturisers, soap substitutes and emollients can be used long-term to maintain skin health, whilst steroid creams and antihistamines can be used during flare-ups. If patients do not respond to such treatments, then oral steroids and antibiotics (in cases of infection) may also need to be considered. Specialist advice from dermatologists and allergists should be sought for further assessment, investigations and subsequent management. If skin surrounding the external auditory canal, nose, oral cavity or eyes is affected, then it may be necessary to contact otorhinolaryngologists and ophthalmologists for an opinion.

7.2 Nose and sinuses

The nasal cavity moistens inhaled air as well as filtering it through the cilia of the nasal mucous membrane with their layer of mucus. The mucus then drains into the pharynx. This activity prevents particles larger than 4–6 microns in diameter from reaching the lungs in inspired air.

Research regarding links between allergic rhinitis and asthma continues. Management therapies should view them as one entity on a continuum, with each having an impact on the other.

Allergic rhinitis affects 20–30% of adults in Europe. Sufferers of allergic disease may get a combination of blocked and runny nose, sinus pain and pressure, excessive post-nasal discharge (which could initially be mucoid and later yellow-green when infected), headache, tiredness and a general feeling of being unwell. These symptoms are not isolated; they can affect surrounding structures such as the ears, throat and eyes, and can even be associated with acid reflux. In severe cases, complications such as sinusitis, infections of the middle ear and nasal polyps may occur, as well as non-specific systemic effects, e.g. fatigue.

A comprehensive history is crucial, with local examination of nose and sinuses including endoscopic examination of nose and post-nasal space. Systemic examination and blood tests appropriate to the history can help to diagnose the causative factor and direct appropriate treatment for the patient.

It is important to identify allergic nasal and sinus disease as, if left untreated, it can lead to infection, making the underlying disease difficult to diagnose. Allergic rhinitis is generally differentiated from non-allergic rhinitis by testing for positive allergenic compounds, for example by skin-prick testing or serum specific IgE testing (a review of the varying forms and causes of rhinitis goes beyond the scope of this book, but further details can be found in *ENT Made Easy*).

Patients with allergic rhinitis are a heterogeneous group of patients; every patient requires tailored treatment, because in some patients rhinorrhoea may be the predominant symptom, whilst others may suffer more from nasal obstruction and sneezing.

Management of allergic rhinitis revolves around allergen avoidance advice, topical medication for symptomatic relief and, where eligibility criteria are met, allergen immunotherapy.

Advice on allergen avoidance is the keystone of the management plan. It should include avoiding peak times of allergen release, planning alternative routes in advance if going outside and using petroleum-jelly-based substances applied to the inner surface at the opening of the nares; this will trap the allergens in the jelly thereby reducing inhalation of allergens.

Routine topical medication is a combination of antihistamines and anti-inflammatories in the form of locally acting steroids. A steroid-based nasal spray or steroid with antihistamine nasal spray should be commenced before the causative season starts and should continue until after the season is over. Correct technique for using topical nasal therapies is key and must be carefully explained and assessed at all levels of care, all the while checking concordance with prescribed medications. This is in addition to ensuring that the shared treatment plan, based on the pathology, is made clear along with duration of treatment and, importantly, how long it will be until the patient starts to feel better.

The atopic march is the name given to the manifestations and progression of allergy-mediated conditions: beginning with eczema, food allergies, allergic rhinitis, nasal polyps and asthma. This march describes how these conditions start from an early age and, if not managed adequately, can go on to peak in adolescence and adulthood.

7.3 Ear

Symptoms of allergy that present at the ear include otitis externa, itch and reduced hearing, which can be due to Eustachian tube dysfunction, serous otitis media or collection of debris in the ear canal. In the case of contact allergy, local reactions to jewellery can be found on the lobule and pinna, the part of the ear that is in contact with the specific allergen.

If the predominant – in some cases the only – symptom is that of itching in the ear, some patients may be using a cotton bud or hair pin to relieve the itch. However, advice should be to avoid doing this, due to the risk of mechanical trauma and subsequent infection. Instead, a medical professional should prescribe the short-term use of a steroid-based ear drop, usually for a week. Allergen avoidance should be advised at the first opportunity. Acute flares may require steroid drops and, if signs of an infection are present, antibiotic drops will be needed in combination. After the acute flare has resolved, short bursts of the steroid drops can be used as and when required. Persistent symptoms should receive specialist review.

Regular use of olive oil drops to act as a moisturiser also helps when commenced at the onset of disease. It helps desquamated skin and wax to fall out and not to irritate the ear lining, thereby avoiding symptomatology and reducing the risk of infection.

In the case of a reduction in hearing or tinnitus because of oedema of the nasal and Eustachian tube lining, treatment in the form of a steroid-based nasal spray or steroid and antihistamine combination nasal spray (with information on technique of use) should be initiated. Patients should know that it can take up to 2 weeks to start noticing signs of improvement. The use of the Otovent balloon twice daily for 1 week, then once daily for another week followed by use as and when required is also a considerable help in Eustachian tube dysfunction. To treat hearing-related symptoms caused by nasal and sinus allergy, patients will need formal hearing assessment such as audio- and tympanograms, use their medications as advised (this may be for a few months), and require specialist follow-up.

In case of local allergenic reaction, for example of the earlobe caused by jewellery, local application of steroid cream to the affected skin with antihistamines orally and locally may be needed. Future avoidance of the metal that triggered the reaction can be advised. If there are further concerns, then clinicians should refer to an allergist for confirmation and further management.

Otitis externa requires a referral to an otorhinolaryngologist, as micro-suction of debris is required initially, along with commencement of antibiotic and steroid-base ear drops that must be reviewed in a specialist ear, nose and throat clinic within a couple of weeks. It is important that patients prevent water from entering the ear during this recovery time.

7.4 Eye

The common symptoms of allergy in an ophthalmological context are itchy, red eyes, epiphora, swelling of the eyelids and a build-up of sticky material around the eye. These symptoms can be very distressing and significantly affect the patient's quality of life. The clinician's role includes a detailed history and examination. The clinical assessment should provide enough information to show whether the disorder could be allergic in nature. Subsequent investigations are usually intended to explore allergic status as opposed to identifying organ-specific variables as appropriate (see *Section 2.3*).

Management principles, again, are avoidance of the allergen (avoiding peak times of allergen release, planning alternative routes in advance if going outside, wearing sunglasses/eye protection) and symptomatic treatment, which can include antihistamine eye drops and a short course of steroid-containing drops in cases of severe allergy. If the disease is difficult to control or severe, ophthalmological advice should be sought sooner rather than later.

7.5 Chest and abdomen

Chest symptoms are covered in *Section 4.4*.

The common symptoms of allergy in the gastrointestinal tract include abdominal pain, vomiting and altered bowel habits. A detailed history with local and systemic examination including nutritional status is important. Referral to a dietitian and specialist advice may be appropriate – *Section 3.7.1* covers this topic.

Chapter 8

Allergy in children

8.1	Clinical assessment of allergy in children	93
8.2	Investigating allergy in children	94
8.3	Food allergy	95
8.4	Asthma	95

The prevalence of allergic diseases and asthma is increasing (current estimates of prevalence are up to 40% in some countries) with greater complexity and severity, especially in children and young adults. This is a worldwide trend and is concerning, given that allergic diseases and asthma are known to negatively affect growth and development, educational attainment, quality of life and social and mental wellbeing. The majority of cases are diagnosed before 7 years of age, with many patients experiencing remission around puberty; however, allergies can return in adulthood.

Common atopic diseases in children are: eczema, asthma, 'hay fever', serous otitis media, allergic rhinitis, allergic rhinoconjunctivitis and food allergies. Acute allergic reaction, in its most lethal form of anaphylaxis, can be due to insect stings or foodstuffs such as nuts. Hospital admissions of children with anaphylaxis are increasing in the UK.

The distribution and pattern of disease changes as the child matures. In the first year of life, it can be difficult to differentiate between an allergy and an infection, or allergies may not present as they typically would in an adult (for example, a child with food allergies may present with rhinitis). Children may suffer from more than one type of allergy at a time; for example, children with rhinitis have a tendency towards asthma, and children with eczema have a tendency to develop rhinitis, food allergy and asthma.

If a RAST (see *Section 2.3*) is positive to HDM and grass pollen at the age of 2 years, it is strongly predictive for later asthma and allergic rhinitis. In a lot of young asthmatic children, HDM is a major allergic component.

Table 8.1 gives a brief overview of some key conditions, including treatments.

Table 8.1 An overview of common allergic diseases in childhood. In all conditions, allergen avoidance should be advocated. Specialist advice should be sought early. Infant: up to 2 years old (yo); child: 2–12 years old; adolescent: 13–18 years old.

Disease	Onset	'Grows out'	Specific treatment considerations
Eczema	Infant	Adolescent	Topical – steroid, antihistamine
Food allergy	Infant	Child (5 yo)	Avoidance with dietitian advice Oral antihistamine
Asthma	Child (3–7 yo)	Adolescent	Inhaled bronchodilators (rescue = beta-blocker, preventer = steroid or combination inhaler)
Allergic rhinitis	Child	Continues to adulthood	Topical – antihistamine and steroid nasal spray Immunotherapy

In most cases multiple systems are involved, so the clinician needs to follow a holistic approach in the treatment of an allergic child. Optimal management of paediatric allergic disease requires medical personnel (general practitioner, paediatrician, allergist and clinical immunologist, specialist e.g. in ENT, respiratory, gastrointestinal, dermatology, ophthalmology), non-medical staff (speech and language therapist, audiologist, school nurse as appropriate) and parents working together for a united plan with clear recommendations. Clear information must be available about the disease itself, its potential emergencies and complications and (with the patient and guardians) side-effects of treatment. Emergency numbers and the general practitioner's details should be up-to-date.

Ensuring the safest environment possible is also very important.

- Adrenaline auto-injectors should be placed at easy access points both at home and school, with a backup at each location, and regularly checked to see if they are in date.
  - This applies to inhalers and nasal sprays too.
  - The teacher or school nurse who looks after the child should know how to use these medications.
- Allergens (e.g. foodstuffs) must be avoided, with the responsible staff routinely checking for this.
  - Contact with the school pet should be avoided in case of animal dander allergy.

Should a child have ear symptoms, they should sit near the front of the class so as to not miss out on learning.

Some children may suffer from multiple atopic conditions and should receive the necessary time out of school to attend their medical appointments. They should be supported in catching up on missed lessons.

8.1 Clinical assessment of allergy in children

A detailed history is of paramount importance; listen carefully to the child (with every possible adjustment/adjunct used to ensure the child can communicate as completely and freely as possible) and to parents or carers. It may be necessary to go into minute detail to gauge the full picture. Collateral information from school may also be helpful.

The common presenting symptoms depend upon the system involved (as shown in *Figure 8.1*). Patients usually have a combination of symptoms; however, parents or carers are usually most concerned by one particular symptom/sign.

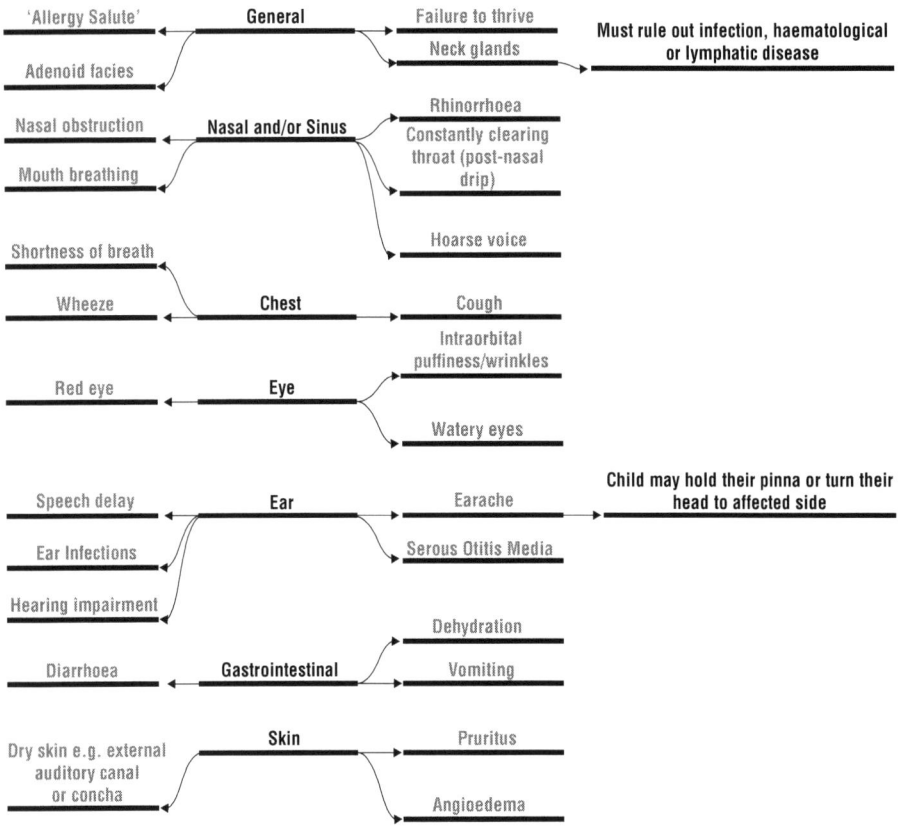

Figure 8.1 Symptoms of organ dysfunction due to allergy.

8.2 Investigating allergy in children

Section 2.3 provides details about allergy tests, but there are limitations for some tests when performed in children suffering from allergy and asthma.

The availability of antihistamines means that, if not directed to withhold these treatments before a test, parents/carers may medicate children, and accordingly tests may produce false negative readings.

The skin-prick test can be performed for specific allergens in over-5 year olds, whilst the RAST blood test can be carried out for under-5 year olds (and if needed, up to 7 year olds). However, there are possible limitations to the use of skin-prick testing, such as needle phobia, non-cooperation during testing, sensitive skin, and the psychological effects on children of seeing a wheal-and-flare reaction on their skin. It should not be attempted in anaphylaxis or in cases of severe reactions.

Peak flow testing can be carried out using a mini-peak flow meter designed for children.

8.3 Food allergy

Food allergy affects 3–6% of children in the developed world. In the UK the incidence of cow's milk allergy is the highest in Europe. In very young children, food allergy is more common than allergies to airborne substances.

The topic is covered in detail in *Sections 3.7.1* and *3.7.3*. Food allergy reaction can present as gastrointestinal, skin, upper or lower respiratory system symptoms in children. Eczema and gastrointestinal symptoms are dominant. It is important to distinguish food allergy from other non-immune-mediated adverse reactions such as food intolerance (often slower onset than IgE-mediated reactions), reaction to ingesting outdated food or a response secondary to metabolic disorder.

The allergen is often a protein component of the food. These water-soluble glycoproteins have varying degrees of resistance to denaturing by heat or acid, therefore may remain intact even after cooking or other treatment. However, a percentage of patients with allergies to the raw form of a foodstuff may be able to tolerate, for example, *boiled* milk or *cooked* eggs.

Simple measures such as a food diary can be a considerable help in identifying the trigger. Skin-prick testing is a rapid and – unless there is a history of anaphylaxis or severe reaction, in which case it should not be carried out – safe method, with a positive test having a sensitivity of approximately 90% but a specificity of only 50%. The negative predictive value generally confirms the absence of IgE-mediated reaction. Where a skin-prick test cannot be done (see *Section 8.2* and the warning above), RAST can be helpful.

Treatment of food allergy relies on allergen avoidance with dietitian input, symptom relief with oral antihistamines and, in some cases, immunotherapy (oral or sublingual). If, for whatever reason, the trigger food is being reintroduced at a later date (it has been reported in some cases that mild food allergies seemingly resolve by school-going age) then it is important that this is done under specialist care.

8.4 Asthma

See *Section 5.4* for details about paediatric asthma.

Index

adaptive immunity, 9
   antibodies, 9
   antibody-antigen complex, 9
   B cells, 9
   cytokines, 10
   immunological memory, 9
   lymphocytes, 9
   T cells, 9
adrenaline, 35
auto-injector, *see* EpiPen
allergen avoidance, for grass and tree
   pollen, 5
allergens, 2
   airborne, 2
   animal, 5
   common, 3
   food, 2, 46
   fungi, 3
   occupational, 2
   pollen, grass and tree, 5
   sensitivity to, 2
allergic bronchopulmonary aspergillosis,
   46
allergic rhinitis, 29, 42
   causative agents, 42
   diagnosis, 42
   management, 43
allergy
   clinical examination in, 22
   diseases to screen for, 21
   to drugs, 50–1
   history-taking in, 20
   to insects, 51–2

allergy – *continued*
   investigations in, 22
   to latex, 51
   management principles in, 78–83; *see*
      also pharmacotherapy in allergy
   of the ear, 44
   of the eye, 41
   of the nose and sinuses, 42–4
   of the respiratory tract, 44–6
   of the skin, 39–41
   presentation in, 20
   routes of exposure, 21
   systemic, 34
allergy types
   cyclic, 17
   fixed, 17
anaphylactoid reaction, 36
   common causes, 36
   diagnosis, 36
   management, 36
anaphylaxis, 34–7
   diagnosis, 34–5
   management, 35
   Resuscitation Council protocol, 36
angioedema, 9, 34, 38
   diagnosis, 38
antibodies, 10
   basic structure, 11
   Fc receptor region, 10
asthma, 55–64
   airflow variability, 59
   categorisation of severity, 63
   complications of, 63–4

asthma – *continued*
    diagnosis, 57–8
    differential diagnoses, 60–2
    management of, 65–76
    pathophysiology, 56
    risk factors for, 57
    stratification of, 57
atopic eczema, 39–40
    diagnosis, 39
    treatment, 40

basophils, 12
blood tests in allergy, 27–8
    ELISA, 28
    RAST, 28
    serum mast-cell tryptase, 28, 34
bronchospasm, 34

C1 esterase inhibitor, 38
challenge tests in allergy, 30
    aspirin challenge, 30
    bronchial provocation challenge, 30
    food challenge, 30
    nasal provocation challenge, 30
clinical examination in allergic patient, 22
cold air as trigger for asthma, 69
compensation, via National Insurance
    (Industrial Injuries) Act 1965, 45
complement system, 7–9
    alternative pathway, 8
    classical pathway, 8
    lectin pathway, 8
    membrane attack complex, 9
conjunctivitis, 41
    treatment, 41
contact dermatitis, 40–1
    nickel sensitivity, 41
cor pulmonale, 45
cross-reactivity, 3
cytokines, 10
cytotoxic T cells, 10, 13, 16

drug allergies, 50–1
    to aspirin, 52–3
    to penicillin, 50

eosinophilia, 28
eosinophils, 7
EpiPen, 20, 35
    in paediatric allergy, 93
exercise-induced bronchoconstriction, 69
    in children, 75
extrinsic allergic alveolitis, *see*
    hypersensitivity pneumonitis

food allergy, 46–50
    common causes, 46–7
    contact allergy, 48–9
    diagnosis, 48
    management, 48
    symptom diary, 48
    see also oral allergy syndrome
fungus, moulds, 3

Gell–Coombs classification, 11
glue ear, *see* otitis media
Graves' disease, 13

histamine, 12
history-taking in allergy, 20–2
    family history, 22
    medication history, 22
house dust, 4
house dust mite, 4
human leukocyte antigen (HLA), 17
hygiene hypothesis, 56
hypersensitivity, 11–17
    Gell–Coombs classification, 11
    type I reaction, 11–13
    type II reaction, 13–14
    type III reaction, 14–15
hypersensitivity pneumonitis, 44
    common causes, 45

immune system, 6–10
    adaptive response, 7
    harmful/non-harmful stimuli, 6
    innate response, 7
    physical barriers, 6
    self/non-self stimuli, 6
immunotherapy, 48

incidence of allergy, 17
inhalers
    spacers, 66
    types, 66
innate immunity, 7
    eosinophils, 7
    self/non-self discrimination, 7
investigations in allergy, 22–30
    blood tests, 27
    nasal inspiratory peak flow, 23
    peak expiratory flow rate, 24
    skin-prick test, 25
    spirometry, 24–5

laboratory tests in allergy, 28–30
    fraction exhaled nitric oxide, 29
    nasal eosinophil smear, 29
    patch test, 29–30

macrophage, 16
management of allergy, 17, 35, 78–83,
    85–9
    organ-specific management, 85–9
    pharmacotherapy, 78–83
    see also specific allergies
management of asthma, 65–76
    aims of, 66
    bronchial thermoplasty, 72
    BTS/SIGN guidelines, 67–8
    immunomodulatory therapy, 72–3
    inhaler types, 66
management of pet allergy, 5
mast cells, 11
mast-cell stabilising agents, 41, 79
monitoring asthma, 73–4
    medication review, 73
    personalised action plan, 73
    symptom review to gauge control, 74
myasthenia gravis, 13

nasal inspiratory flow (peak), 24
nasal inspiratory rate (peak), 24
nasal polyposis, 44

occupational asthma, 59

opsonin, 8
oral allergy syndrome, 49
organ-specific management of allergy,
    85–9
    ear, 88
    eye, 89
    nose and sinuses, 86–8
    skin, 86
otitis externa, 89
otitis media, 44

paediatric allergy, 91–5
    clinical assessment, 93–4
    common atopic disease, 92
    investigations, 94–5
    symptoms of organ dysfunction, 94
    to foods, 95
    to house dust mite, 92
paediatric asthma, 74–6
    BTS/SIGN Guidelines for Management,
        76
    management of, 75–6
    wheeze phenotypes, 75
pharmacotherapy in allergy, 78–83
    anticholinergics, 82
    antihistamines, 78
    corticosteroids, 80
    decongestants, 80
    immunotherapy, 82
    mast-cell stabilisers, 79
    side-effects of drug treatment, 79, 80,
        81, 82
pharmacotherapy in asthma, 67–72
    anticholinergics, 71
    beta-2 agonists, 67, 69
    combination therapy (LABA and ICS),
        69
    corticosteroids, 69–70
    cromones, 72
    leukotriene receptor agonists, 71
    side-effects of drug treatment, 70, 71
    theophylline, 71–2
pollen fruit syndrome, 49
presentation of allergy, 20
pseudopodia, 27

radiological imaging in allergy, 31

serum-specific IgE testing, 42
Severe Asthma Registry (UK), 72
skin-prick test, 25, 42, 49
    axon reflex, 26
    equipment required, 26
    results, 26–7
    wheal and flare response, 26–7
spirometry, 24–5
    features of with asthma, 59
    FEV_1, 25
    FVC, 25
    with bronchodilator, 25
    with exercise, 25
sulphite sensitivity, 52
systemic lupus erythematosus (SLE), 9, 15

T helper cells, 10
T regulatory cells, 10
thymus, 10
type I hypersensitivity, 11, 34
    early and late phase, 12
type II hypersensitivity, 13
    diseases resulting, 13
type III hypersensitivity, 14
    diseases resulting, 15
type IV hypersensitivity, 16
    diseases resulting, 16

venom allergies, 51

wheal and flare, in skin-prick testing,
    26–7